Friday Forever

Memoirs of Madness

T0132718

Friday Forever
Memoirs of Madness

SUSAN BRADLEY SMITH

Senior Lecturer in English and Creative Writing
Melbourne, Australia

Forewords by

JANETTE TURNER HOSPITAL

Carolina Distinguished Professor Emerita

Department of English

University of South Carolina

and

JILL GORDON

General Practitioner

Honorary Associate Professor, Medical Humanities

Centre for Values, Ethics & the Law in Medicine

University of Sydney

Radcliffe Publishing
London • New York

Radcliffe Publishing Ltd
33–41 Dallington Street
London
EC1V 0BB
United Kingdom

www.radcliffepublishing.com
Electronic catalogue and worldwide online ordering facility.

British Library Cataloguing in Publication Data

A catalogue record for this book is available from the British Library.

ISBN-13: 978 184619 036 0

The paper used for the text pages of this book
is FSC® certified. FSC (The Forest Stewardship
Council®) is an international network to promote
responsible management of the world's forests.

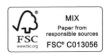

Typeset by Pindar NZ, Auckland, New Zealand
Printed and bound by TJI Digital, Padstow, Cornwall, UK

Cover photograph used with the permission of Walker Photography & Design

Contents

Foreword

In the middle of the journey of his life, Dante *came to himself within a dark wood where the straight way was lost.* So *savage and harsh and dense* was that thicket of grief and anomie that he had to 'touch bottom', to descend deep into the inferno of his depression before he could write his way out. He had to *know* it, explore its murkiest recesses, analyze it. His guide was Virgil, poet of a prior literary work of dispossession, dislocation and loss. In the *Divine Comedy*, Dante rewrote the script of private trauma (exile, unrequited love) and gave himself – on a cosmic scale – the happy ending that eluded him in life. He was neither the first nor the last to turn inward chaos into a work of self-interrogation and art.

Many centuries before Dante, the lone survivor of an annihilated community spoke of trauma so catastrophic that only poetry could contain it. *He who has felt it knows how cruel a companion is sorrow to him who has no beloved protectors* . . . and yet the 'Wanderer' in this Anglo-Saxon lament groped his way, line by poetic line, to a stoic serenity. 'That is why poetry exists', Susan Bradley Smith reminds us in her memoir, 'to speak the unspeakable'. But the unspeakable is like molten lava in a stoppered volcano: it cannot be contained; it erupts; it insists on finding its way out. There is a long literary tradition of constructing a ladder of words and using it to climb from anguish to peace of mind. That tradition is bequeathed to all as testament, consolation, and rescue route. Susan's memoir inherits and contributes to this distinguished lineage.

Happiness is beneficial for the body, noted Marcel Proust, *but it is grief that develops the powers of the mind.* Multiple griefs battered Susan like a string of cyclones, one following on the heels of another: the break-up of a marriage, the near-death of a child, the recurrence of a rare genetic disorder in two children, major geographic displacement. All these matters are right at the top of the stress scale and are indicators of risk of clinical depression, but they are also – in some sense – random and impersonal, experienced by many. Add to these body blows an act of deliberate malice: a crude, vicious, intentionally personal and grossly unjust attack on academic integrity. The result in emotional terms is equivalent to the onrush of Katrina on the vulnerable levees of New Orleans. One of the many things that this memoir demonstrates is the inadequacy of academia's response to egregious violations of professional ethics. Legal bases are covered as a matter of course and the accusations against Susan were officially found to be false and malicious; but acknowledging the mayhem that ensues from breaches in ethical conduct is something all too often ignored by academic institutions. Actual intervention to curtail the viral spread of slander seems to be quite beyond the moral will of university administrations.

What happened might have destroyed Susan's career and rendered her seriously dysfunctional. For a time, that is exactly what occurred. But Susan did what Dante did, what intellectuals and artists have always done: she observed the dark places with an acute and unsparing eye, she analyzed, she wrote her way out. She has written with rigorous honesty and witty self-deprecation. She has also written a memoir about the ethics of writing a memoir. Her interrogation of the genre of confessional writing is as scrupulous as her self-interrogation and she has followed the prescription laid down by Yeats:

Now that my ladder's gone,
I must lie down where all the ladders start
In the foul rag and bone shop of the heart.

Janette Turner Hospital
Carolina Distinguished Professor Emerita
Department of English
University of South Carolina
Columbia, SC
April 2011

vii

Foreword

This is a crazy book. I wish it had been around 30 years ago. That's how long I've been working as a GP specialising in psychotherapy. And that's how long I've been wishing for a crazy book about postnatal depression, instead of all the sensible ones. So many of my patients have plunged out of sensible, ordered, well-managed, intelligent lives into the mess of motherhood and found themselves overwhelmed.

This book takes one unique experience and asks the reader *'Could it be, could it have been, like this for you too?'* And I know that the answer, from many of the women that I have seen, would be *'Yes – a lot of it was just like that. The details are different, but the guilt, the regret, the bleakness, the ruminations, the obsessions, and the other mad thoughts were all there for me too. Thank you for telling me that I'm not alone.'*

'But what about the fact that I can't think, can't focus, can't remember anything – can't really function?' A single sentence captures one of the characteristic experiences of depression:

> *'I opened the newspaper one morning and found I could not read it.'*

As frightening as that sounds, this is actually a reassuring book. Not only for women who have felt like this, but for the doctors and other therapists who believe that the way back to sanity can be traced in a genuine effort to understand, as much as any person can understand, another person who is suffering. There are lots of 'evidence-based psychological therapies' (EBPTs) for mental illness – a Google search uncovers 73,000 entries and their inevitable acronyms. EBPTs have their place; after all, the evidence says so and I don't doubt it. But if that's all there is, then we might as well all give up on any vision of a crazy, enriching, exciting, challenging, accepting, engaging, mind-expanding world. We might as well all be sensible, cautious, risk-averse, single-minded and brain-dead.

I'm reminded of Margaret Thatcher talking to *Women's Own Magazine* in 1987:

> '*And, you know, there is no such thing as society. There are individual men and women, and there are families ... people must look to themselves first.*'

What Susan says in reply is roughly this: there *is* such a thing as society and we can't live without it. There *are* times when we are unable to look after ourselves or to look after someone we love who is in terrible danger when we don't know what to do, and we need help.

Susan knew what she needed and what she lacked:

> '*I would sit there and think about how I recently read something about T S Eliot and his theory of the "auditory imagination", and how a poem can communicate something real to us before we even understand it, and wondering if therapists can listen to patients like this, in this special kind of way. I would will them that special talent, as I sat, choking on my despair.*'

A sense of society starts with a 'special kind of way' of listening to one another. It's a message, not just for therapists, but for anyone who wants to be part of a society. It starts with being quiet and paying attention. It just happens to be particularly important when one is paying attention to another person who is ill or frightened or sad.

Along with that important message is the same message that William Styron conveyed in *Darkness Visible*. Love is the key. For Susan it was the discovery of her capacity to find the place 'where love for my husband and love for children collide ... The grace of that shaking love, that is what shook my depression away'.

Friday Forever is a gift for anyone who has struggled with the illness caused by depression, anyone who has wanted to help a family member or friend, any health professional who wants to have a better understanding of the patient's experience of illness and anyone who simply wants to know more about what it means to be human.

Jill Gordon
General Practitioner
Honorary Associate Professor, Medical Humanities
Centre for Values, Ethics & the Law in Medicine
University of Sydney
April 2011

About the author

Susan Bradley Smith was educated at the University of New South Wales and University of New England, and began her writing life as a theatre and music journalist in Sydney and later London. Widely published as a literary and theatre historian and creative writer, her latest book, *supermodernprayerbook* (Salt, 2010) was shortlisted for the Kenneth Slessor Poetry Prize. Recent publications include *Griefbox and other Plays*, a selection of her own plays, and her first collection of poetry, *Marmalade Exile*. Susan has research interests in 21st century literature, lifewriting, and medical humanities (bibliotherapy). She lives in Melbourne and Lennox Head.

Acknowledgements

Diana Cooper once wrote in a letter to Evelyn Waugh that 'Meg is back at school so I can start work again on the account of my lunacy', and this is what writing this book has felt like, one big wait for the children to go back to school before I could turn to face this 'dark material'. This has meant that I've kept an awful lot of people waiting a long time, most patiently of all perhaps Gillian Nineham. Thanks are due to her for commissioning this book in the first place, and her unfailing support and friendship over the years. Others kept waiting include the usual family suspects (who as I write this are at the beach sans me, as usual), most of all my husband James, and our children. This book is dedicated to Scarlet because of all our children I believe I was most 'absent' with her due to illness, and I'd like to acknowledge her and her siblings' strident understanding of the business of ill health, of writing and writers, and thank them for their questions and permissions. I would also like to thank other family and friends who thought that it was worth writing about this subject, and encouraged me: George, Gabrielle, Leonie, Susan, Rachael, Jackie, Amber, Barb, Julie, Graeme, Therese, Nettie, Donna, Jo, Alan, and everyone else, with special thanks to the women who shared their stories, and were always there for me. This book is of course a medical memoir, about my long romp with postnatal depression, a time when I was so far away from the idea of my favourite day of the week, 'Friday', it felt like the week hadn't yet been invented. Obviously, a story about depression is a story about collisions and collapses, and about the lack of accord that happens when we are a long way away from health. So I would also like to thank everyone (especially Ian) involved in my healthcare, even if things did not always go so well. Thanks also are due to Julian Croft and Peter Porter for permission to quote from their poetry, and the editors of the literary and poetry journals and collections where some of the poems, and versions of chapters and extracts first appeared: *Text*; *Australian Family Physician*; *Transnational Literature*; *Salt Magazine*; *Lost and Found*; and *Over There: Poems from Singapore and Australia*.

For Scarlet Rebel

Epigraph

'Life's tea party:
someone brings in the tray
and the cloth is pulled away . . .'

Julian Croft, 'Concentration', *Ocean Island*

'Don't fall down now
You will never get up
Don't fall down now'

Everclear, 'Strawberry', *Sparkle and Fade*

Chapter 1

What I didn't know: life in topsy-turvy land

Once upon a time my favourite writer was the English children's author Enid Blyton. She was the first person who defined 'daring' for me, and the adventures of her 'Famous Five' and 'Secret Seven' permanently distinguished my lust for life. Most impressionably, like the characters in her 'Faraway Tree', I too believed that atop the tallest magic tree in the forest there was an ever-changing world, and you never knew what the children would find each different day they visited – Land of the Slaps one day, Land of Birthdays the next – nor what joys or terrors they might encounter. No matter what happened though, they always made it home safely for supper, and to help mother. This, I thought, was the proper metaphor for life, one full of robust play coupled with responsible duty. Imagine my surprise then to find myself one day stuck atop the tree in topsy-turvy land, with the cloud having moved on, and no foreseeable escape route. Nothing was normal, everyone was crazy, and so it seemed was I. And that was that. How does one write their way out of this?

I grew up in a working-class family in regional New South Wales, Australia, and knew about droughts and farms and how to avoid kangaroos whilst driving at sunset. Moving around, I also came to know about sunburn and beaches and sandbanks and rips. Later I learnt about inner-city Sydney and independent theatre and pub rock when I became the first in my seventh-generation Australian family (yes – convict ancestry) to attend university. As soon as I graduated, in 1986, I took myself and my education and a suitcase full of Australian beer to London and never properly came back, until I found myself married and pregnant. I would be fibbing if I said that every single moment had been like my childhood fantasy of 'Land of the Birthdays', but overall I felt blessed to be living a life of my own choosing, professionally satisfied working in publishing and education, and was grateful for all the glee of my London life. In summary, one hell of a charmed existence.

Late in 1996 I fell pregnant with my eldest daughter, and in early 1997 it seemed prudent to return home. Soon after the birth I found myself wandering around the craggy cliff top of one of Sydney's most beautiful beaches contemplating suicide. Lots of things happened during that first year of motherhood, but not that: I never jumped. Instead, I stayed away from tempting heights, and tried to get on with things, in my shambolic way. A few years later, somehow I had migrated back to England, commenced an academic career, divorced, remarried, and my second daughter was born in 2002. Then, the place I loved most in the world, my hometown of London, suddenly became a quarry of despair when my baby daughter was diagnosed with a rare medical condition. Our world collapsed. It was a crazy time, and I made mad and bad decisions that I am still paying for, that we are all still paying for. And when my son was born the following year, also to be diagnosed with MCADD, and the sky moved as close as possible to earth without actually suffocating me, I took this huge weight with me and flew it back to Australia.

Soon afterwards, I had a nervous breakdown. It was not until very late, too late, in the recovery game, when one of my doctors said the words 'postnatal depression' to me, that I even began to be able to start making sense of the barb-wired mess of my life. So much pain, and such extensive ignorance. We live in such smooth, modern, safe worlds, women like me. Educated. Privileged. Loved. Medical provision on tap. Logistically, it seems impossible that my illness could have been so long, so significant, and so undetected. And I nearly lost myself to it, not to mention the costs that linger on for all of us. That, this, is my story. And my story would have been oh so very different, would no doubt have remained under-cover forever, if not for a series of unfortunate events, for whose intervention I am now forever grateful. That is why the story must begin not with the birth of my first child, but first with the incident that brought me to my knees. Only then can I take you back to all those other dangerous, crumbling, sandstone cliff tops. This is a book about postnatal depression. I am going to be confessing things to you that I have not told my doctors, have not told my husband, or family, and certainly not your average casual acquaintance. I am not entirely sure I want my children to be reading about all this either; that is, if they ever fancy the chore of knowing their mother better. But I can't tell you my story, which is really a tale about getting sick, and what makes women sick, and how women might heal, without broaching some taboo subjects, which will hopefully enlighten, so I have to ignore any apprehension. Why me? I often wondered this. Why do any of us suffer from depression – you can't but help pondering why the bad things that happen to you, well, happen to *you*. But, happen they did. I had a nervous breakdown, and was signed off work. Some excruciating time later, I was diagnosed with postnatal depression, amongst other things. I need to begin by telling a story about how fear came into my life, big time, and took away my sanity. So, as the story opens, I am already a mother of three young children, aged 7, just 2, and almost 1. The setting is regional Australia. I was working full-time as a university lecturer, and my husband was seeking work whilst acting as primary caregiver to our children.

APRIL 2004, LENNOX HEAD, AUSTRALIA

'There she goes, my beautiful girl'. The music on the car radio was doing its loud, good thing. It was a perfect North Coast winter's day, not shying away from its subtropical promise. Not even a wetsuit needed for this morning's surf. Driving up through the bush from the beach on my way to work, inland, to a small regional Australian city, you can see the scars of white settlement – sugarcane on ancient marshes, dairy cattle ghosting what was once deep-cedared forests, that once-upon-a-time helped build Sydney and Melbourne. *I love this song.* No kids in the back to referee, no one to moan about my singing. Higher. The sound level would surely disqualify my ears from any purposeful service. Even when he was only a medical student, in the early 1980s, my brother would responsibly stand up the back at rock gigs all over Sydney – 'I'll need my ears to detect a heart murmur one day' – but while I agreed with and admired him, I moved away, lower, closer to the front, closer to the boom, closer, always, to the noise, to harm. I turned the radio up another notch. I was going to be late for my 3 o'clock lecture. It was 2:35, and the university was still 20 minutes drive away, not even considering the parking, the walking, the 'where are my lecture notes?' time consumption. 'There she goes, my beautiful girl'. I drove faster, pushing 100 kmph in an 80 zone. *What a great song.* I am, suddenly, happy. Mad with it. Thrilled to have finally found the right song for baby Scarlet's funeral. It was an exact fit with her: passionate, pumping, rocking, poignant. Just like her 2-year-old self. I could see the whole scene in front of me, as I curved the road into Lismore: my husband and my brother and the small, desperate coffin, leaving the church. Righteous. Me. Unable to look. Not crying. For once, not speaking at a public family event. Not saying anything. Serenity. It was over. Rituals to abate pain.

Driving way too fast, I began to sob as the song ended. What was I thinking? I hated myself. I braked, slowing down to a widowly 60 kmph. What *was* I thinking? Driving like that? A mother of three children. Hooning past the corner, THE corner, that very same corner on this exact piece of road where my very own boyfriend and best friend had both died. Twenty-three years ago. And my little psychodrama story to amuse myself whilst speeding – what was that all about? Sick woman. My stuff of fantasy, delivered unbidden, has revolted me my whole life long. *Scarlet is not dead.* Scarlet was not dead. Scarlet is not dead. Scarlet did not die. She woke up from her coma 19 months ago, and despite all the hospitalisations since, has remained bold, strong, gorgeous, and very much alive.

'That was Nick Cave and the Bad Seeds with "There she goes my beautiful world"'. I turned the radio off. I slowed down even more. I was going to be late for 120 students. A lecture on *The Merchant of Venice.* They would wait. I would be very sorry. I would make up for it, razzle dazzle. Soon I would drive home again. Run my babies on the beach. Feed them. Bed them. Kiss them too long, especially Scarlet, me with my silent sorries. Drink large quantities of wine. Mark essays. Drink more wine. *In sooth I know not why I am so sad.* 'My beautiful world.' My beautiful girl. My girl.

I get it wrong, all the time. But does anyone ever notice? Especially if you sing loud enough? What I did not know, on that beautiful day, was that I was close, very close, to a nervous breakdown that had been waiting for me for a long time. Later, I would learn that I had been suffering from postnatal depression on and off since the birth of my first child in September 1997. Life and its trying circumstances had left me undiagnosed and constantly struggling. Shortly, I was about to feel that very light touch of the straw that breaks a camel's back. Something was about to go terribly wrong at work, and in the aftermath everything I had been trying so valiantly to suppress would surface into a full-blown kind of madness.

How did all this happen, how did it come to this? Is illness ever a gift? Is recovery ever complete? What if, at certain points in history, I had made different decisions: could I have avoided all this pain, no matter how edifying it might now feel? How far back into the past do you have to go to try and understand yourself, and your vulnerabilities? This story tries to answer all of those questions, as honestly and intelligently as I can. It was horrid being mad, and for the most part my experience of the medical and therapeutic processes of healing was not altogether a happy one. So this book is a candid account of those times, of illness and recovery, but it asks a lot of hard questions about women and mental health and the doctor–patient relationship, hoping that my telling will ease that journey for others. To quote from Ian McEwan's novel *Black Dogs*, where one of his characters declares, 'I have taken a number of liberties, the most flagrant of which has been to recount certain conversations never intended for record', I should warn that I also feel that telling my own story is some kind of trespass. I have thought hard about the ethics of memoirs – who owns the story, when so many people inhabit the narrative? – and my own personal decision is that I have laid down my weapons, and if people want to shoot me while I am praying a prayer of intercession for the well-being of women, then so be it. So – how did it all begin? How did I end up in the shooting gallery?

A few short months earlier, I had been safe in London. In December 2003, we had just celebrated our second Christmas in our new home, recently renovated to accommodate our growing family. Here I am, dramatising my real life, explaining our decision to leave, as though to tell it in the first person I might catch on fire. The 'her' is me; the 'him' is James, my second husband. This was one of those moments that changed our lives.

SCENE I

An office in a loft of a renovated Victorian home in a dodgy part of East London. Christmas. Decorations. Laptops. Carols playing in the background. Books. Desks. A futon.

HIM   Are you going to send it?

HER   No. I don't know.

HIM   Go on. I'm sick of this shite weather.

HER   How about. Some sex. Maybe.

HIM   Send it. Go on. You know they want you.

HER   I've been there, you know. Australia. Mate. Childhood. Hello? Regional Australia is something you know nothing about. Herr Professor.

HIM   No. Of course not. Silly me. Convict historian that I am. Nothing to know is there? Silly bloody me. Look. Surely they know how to play cricket?

HER   Shut up. Plus. You can't surf. I'm not sure you can even actually swim properly. You do realise that you'll be the only male in Lennox Head more than 4 years old who can't surf. If I get the job. That is. If they do want me. Because we'll have to live at the beach. I would never, ever, live in Lismore. Again. Not after. Well.

HIM   Bloody terrible idea. The beach. Rotten. Send it.

HER   What will you do?

HIM   Jesus wept. What will I do? Same as bloody usual. Pretend to write books and hang around waiting to take one of the children to hospital.

HER   What?

HIM   I mean it.

HER   Full-time Daddy?

HIM   Yes.

HER   You'll have every Mum in the village after you. You and your naked self. Darling. Australian women are very untrustworthy you know. Sluttish lot, we are. Damned whores and all.

HIM   Quite right.

HER   You want to look after the babies? Seriously?

HIM   Yes. Now push the bloody button and come to bed and make me another one.

HER   What if? What if I can't. Look. I don't really like my family that much. For a start. You know. What if –

He undresses her.

HIM   We'll come back. We can always come back. We'll rent the house out, that way, if and when we want to come back, to come back to live in our delightfully bankrupt borough, in our shabby but stately falling-down home, a block from gun mile, around the corner from the only hospital in England that has a police station attached to it. We can come back and return to weekending in Brighton complaining about the water quality or ducking over to France on a wine run, staring at the extremely stimulating interior of the Eurostar whilst Scarlet screams all the way to Calais. And back. To Hackney. 3pm nightfalls. Two hours plus commute to work. Nannies that milk you dry in between getting deported. The River Lea and all its polluted glory to row upon. The greasy spoon as Saturday breakfast. Any time you want. We can come back. Two hundred pound weekly grocery shops, the M25, Heathrow on Friday nights, parents that –

HER   All right. Enough.

She sends the email.

HER   I personally have nothing against a bacon and egg sandwich on Saturday morning watching the houseboats go by. You bloody bully. Pommy bastard.

He holds her. They are both naked.

HER   What about your girls? Your other babies? We can't leave them behind. Can we?

SILENCE

SCENE II

The master bedroom, two weeks later. Dawn. She opens the curtains and waves across the narrow street to a neighbour doing the same. She is on the phone, and breastfeeding.

HER   Sure. OK. Yes. Look, that's OK. I'd prefer it if she wasn't on sab-batical. No. Yes. No. Yes, a quick start is what I want.

Silence

HER   I understand. Yes. No. I don't regard it as a demotion. I'll be perfectly happy. Yes. I'll do that. I'll wait for your email. Thank you again. Yes. It really is very kind if you to offer me the job.

Laughs

HER Thank you. Thank you very much. OK. Yes. Goodbye. Goodnight.

Hangs up. Hums. Feeds.

HER Fancy a home among the gumtrees then little one?

Another baby, off, cries. She looks out at the snow falling.

TO BE CONTINUED

So that was that. James had been unemployed for too long. I loved our new home in a run-down part of Hackney, which we had only just finished restoring, and planting a garden, to raise the children in. It was big enough to host friends and most importantly family – James's two daughters from his first marriage lived in Edinburgh with their mother, but all three of them were regular visitors, as was my eldest daughter's father – ex-husband Matthias, who came often from Germany to spend time with Ulrike. Three adults, five children, the weekending grandfather, endless stray Australians, and all the rest, the house was for all of us to call home. I was very happy, but what do you do when things become unsustainable? When husbands can't find jobs and children are too often in hospital and mortgage payments are missed? The reality of our life at this time was that our income did not cover our basic needs, and that we had two children under 18 months old who had a rare metabolic disorder that (then) demanded constant vigilance and care from us.

Well, what happens is this. You make a decision from a tight corner, and imagine a better future. You believe that accepting a job in a regional university and living in the country rather than the city will be good for your bank balance, and will allow your children to grow up in 'paradise' at a beach seven miles long. You believe that you can talk everyone you love in Edinburgh and England and Germany into joining you on this odyssey. You believe a lot of things that really, deep inside, you know to be some kind of mad fiction, but in the absence of better advice (any advice, really, except from the children's specialist consultant at Great Ormond Street Hospital for Children, who said 'choose safely') and in the grip of postnatal depression you get on a plane and that is that. It all seems so romantic. In the days, weeks, and years to come, I have barely paused in my long regret of that decision.

It all might have been different. The decision may not have been the soundest one, but it was made completely unsafe by a fate from left field that caught us all out. Me, especially me, who needed to be the strongest, and was not. Me, the Australian who should know her own country, the mother who had to work to feed the family; the tired, sick woman who fell down one day and found she could not get up. This is what happened, six months after coming back to Australia to begin a new life.

JULY 2005, LISMORE, AUSTRALIA

I was very frightened. Some months earlier, a postgraduate student had accused me of plagiarism.

Dear Susan

Forgive this email. I'm sorry, but you are my supervisor, and I have to know. Are you a plagiarist, as she says? I suppose you know what I mean. Please phone me.

Yours, truly . . .

This is how I found out I was being accused, from a 'friendly' student email, by one of my own postgraduates. Not from my colleagues, who were already investigating me without having informed me, which was a clear breach of university protocol. I had been under the hammer since I arrived back in Australia and began this job. There were only two permanent staff on the creative writing programme, myself and my colleague who was on sabbatical. So, I was on my own with a bevy of postgraduates who were working as casual tutors. On top of my long commute, I had three new courses to teach, deliver, and coordinate. I rarely left work before 7pm. James was battling on his own with three children through my long absences, and dealing with my increasing exhaustion as best he could.

Following the accusation, I was at first numb, then sick with worry during the investigation period. After my name was cleared, I did not begin to get angry until some time later, when I felt my own health and my entire family's well-being and livelihood threatened by the unresolved nature of the situation. Some misguided person was wrongly attacking me, was still attacking me, and the costs were enormous. For an academic and writer, being accused of plagiarism can permanently damage one's career. The stain of the accusation, no matter how the story unwinds, is forever there. It wasn't really a straw then that broke my back, but a large slab of concrete dropped from on high, all over my too fragile (sick) self. Could I recover and protect myself and my family? I just wanted it to stop, I wanted that woman to cease her vendetta against me, and allow me to protect our decision to live this life.

How had this craziness begun? On 'the day of my downfall', in a scenario that felt somewhat like *Alice in Wonderland* being read backwards, James and Scarlet ended up in the small local hospital, whereas I had been told by the ambulance man to go to the base hospital further away in Lismore. When I arrived, I was instructed to wait, rather than drive back down to Ballina, as they were just stabilising Scarlet before moving her either up to Lismore, or flying her to Brisbane. They kept telling me they'd know any minute. I kept vomiting. The sister in emergency was wonderful. *Haven't you got somewhere you'd rather wait? I'll phone you immediately. You know, there's nothing you can do here. Aside from vomit in my bathroom.* I took advice, deciding to go and wait it out in my office, as the university was just around the corner and down the hill.

Yes. I knew too well about preparing for the long haul of Scarlet's hospitalisations. I went to do just that. Even though I had already left a message that I wouldn't be able to make my 9am class (a three-hour seminar) I suddenly became extremely focused on this problem. Did my message get through? I had more than likely left it with the university gardener for all I knew. How bad it must look, not turning up for this advanced theory class. What would they do without me? So, mobile in pocket, I grabbed my notes which I had been collating on the bathroom floor last night as James I had been taking turns to nurse Scarlet through her vomiting fits, and ran off down the corridor to make my apologies in person.

When I arrived in the seminar room I was surprised but gratified to note that rather than finding a room full of stranded students a postgraduate student had stepped in unasked and was leading discussions. I quickly apologised for my no-show. Then, as I had started to shake and could tell I was about to cry, I smartly left, thanking the tutor and handing her my notes. These were the very notes that she soon used to fabricate her claims of plagiarism. I did not go to my office, but ran to my car and drove straight back to the hospital. Scarlet had arrived but I had not been phoned. Typical. But Scarlet was going to be OK. While we there, sorting out her world, mine was being poisoned by the person I have come to refer to as 'that woman'. While Scarlet was being cannulated, 'that woman' was swiftly and maliciously fabricating a story, fully designed to bring me to my knees. In time I came to believe that if I did not prove her wrong, and defend my innocence, Scarlet would die. 'That woman' and her crusade against me was a test sent to me by the gods, a metaphor for defending my family against evil so that my children could prosper. Sound mad? Maybe. But ask any mother who has lived most of her life with men who don't earn an income how precious her job is, how essential it is to keep her family safe, warm, fed, gifted, and how she'd feel if someone was threatening that. Just ask her what she'd think. Her answer might sound a tad crazed too.

When it was all over, and I was proved innocent, the victory for me meant that Scarlet would live. That was all that mattered. Like the shark that every surfer has seen but needs to believe does not spell their demise, I had thought myself protected by the certainty that another set of waves to catch was the purpose of life: keep on keeping on. The statistics are on your side, cars kill, not sharks. Ignore the sharks. Shortly after seeing Scarlet safely to the firm shores and hard sands of low tide, I fell over, fully, into the shark-infested waters of a nervous breakdown. Not without some drama for all involved. Drama or melodrama? Three short paragraphs: that's all it has taken to summarise a life drama that nearly resulted in a gravestone.

During the months since the dismissed allegations when my accuser's claims against me were proved wrong, as borne out by the committee's investigations, her outrageous conduct surrounding the making of these allegations nevertheless had damaged my reputation, not to mention my health. And, she would not give up: when the university found against her, she refused to accept their findings and continued her public campaign to destroy my reputation which involved lobbying students and staff, and selling her story to the national press. That was not a good day for me, when that story made front-page news. I went into work to find one of my senior academic colleagues distributing copies of the newspaper to one and all in our faculty. Friendly. Eventually, I had had enough, and asked the management to do something to support me, to make this all stop. I just wanted to work, free of bullying and accusations and slanders. I just wanted it all to end.

And today, I thought it would, I thought that this meeting would be a chance for them to thank me for sticking it, coming to work every day and doing a fine job, despite the shame and humiliation and the emotional taxation that results from such allegations.

Today, I thought, it would begin to be over. But something intuitive warned me that things might not be that simple. As I walked across campus for a meeting with the acting vice chancellor, and my faculty dean, I meandered down the ramp crossing the small gully, and passed through a patch of rainforest that yesterday had revealed a python as nature's gatekeeper between all who worked in our building, and the car park with the cars beyond. Some people walked on, unperturbed, others took the long way around. Today, I wouldn't mind seeing that big snake again. Maybe I could take it along with me to the meeting. I needed someone on my side. Winter. Not a season to be jolly.

This meeting had been called because I had let it be known that in my opinion I felt the university was not supporting me sufficiently in a time of crisis. In particular, that the woman who had maliciously slandered me and accused me of being a plagiarist, although investigations had completely exonerated me, and she had been disciplined, was still a PhD candidate in our school, and continued to send me threatening emails (and circulated continual allegations of plagiarism to what seemed to me like half the world – certainly she was contacting UK colleagues). She had already been dismissed as a tutor (not for her allegations, but for her conduct surrounding the allegations) but was still only a few doors down from me in the corridor of our very small university. Rustling infantry. *You know she's a plagiarist.* As you might imagine, this 'high drama' was very preoccupying. Sick children at home? Ignore this. My own inability to sleep or stop crying all night? Don't tell anyone. That comforting children that still needed feeding every two hours during the night left me in a robotic relationship with them? Don't mention it to anyone, anyone, that I could feel no love for them, only duty. Older daughter having problems with settling at school? Comparatively inconsequential (how shameful this is to write). Husband talking too much about the women he was meeting at playgroup? Pour him another drink. Until I slayed the monster at work, everything was under threat. First things first. Was I sure that I was being treated poorly, or had I completely lost perspective? As I walked to the meeting, I recalled the first moment of terror. Not for the first time, I asked myself why I cared so much about my professional reputation. The answer was always the same. If I work, I can protect my family. If I don't, we lose everything. But had I given up breastfeeding my babies for this rubbish life, where I was unsafe and abused at work? No. I had not.

This was my worry today, on my way to this important meeting:

that the university was (rightly as it turned out) worried about my accuser's litigious conduct, and was therefore not keen to discipline her further. Consequently, in my opinion, I felt that it was being privately hoped that I would simply suffer this abuse stoically and not make further 'trouble'. Because, obviously, complaining about students in a customer-driven market is always a bother. Was I right? Was I collateral damage? All I knew for certain was that they were sitting on my complaint, and had been for an unreasonably long time. A complaint that had been lodged, in fact, on the advice of the university solicitor. *If you don't give us the evidence, how can we do anything?* Why does evidence always feel so dirty? When I formally lodged my complaint I claimed that, despite the allegations against me being heard and dismissed by everyone from the appropriate university committee to the ombudsman, my accuser was still decrying me. According to her, I remained and always would be a plagiarist, and did not deserve my position as an academic. She was routinely sending me emails, reminding me that I was a plagiarist, threatening me with legal action, and demanding that I issue proclamations that I had read her draft PhD thesis and would never publish that material under my name. No chance of that ever happening, I can promise you! (Sometimes I think that might explain this whole sordid ordeal: she never appreciated my critical appraisal of her draft thesis – in fact, she never responded to my extensive annotated commentary, representing some 15 hours or more work – which is extraordinary conduct for a student. Her next communication with me was to accuse me of plagiarism!)

Every morning, I left my babies in a crazed rush to get to work. Hunter was only 5 months old when we came home to Australia. Sure, every morning, I walked with him in a backpack as I trawled the long, lonely beach, but it was not the surf or his gorgeous gurgles that I heard. The soundtrack in my mind was an endless composition of self-righteousness. I needed it: every morning, when I arrived at work, when I opened my email, there it was, today's fresh rant against me. Insulting me. Making me ill. When I hesitantly lodged a complaint about this harassment, my complaint was not dealt with by due university procedures. In fact, I received no response at all. I had to chase things up, endlessly. Later, I discovered the reason for this 'silence' was that the woman in question was in the middle of levelling serious complaints against the university for the manner in which she perceived they had handled her complaints against me. She was, indeed, a ticking bomb, and the university was worried about a lot more things than my professional reputation, wounded ego or mental health. To my great cost.

When I complained about my complaint not being dealt with, the rejoinder was extraordinary. I was sent a 17-page letter in response to my complaint against this student for her continual harassment (remember, a complaint that the university solicitor had insisted that I lodge) by the university's external workplace lawyers, informing me of how supportive the university was. It was an extraordinary document. Full of 'quotes' from meetings that I attended but with no witnesses present, no minutes, yet this legal letter offered these reports of meetings as evidence of kindness, and fulsome management. Such 'support' had left me terrified, and my own (now privately engaged) solicitor champing at the bit to retaliate. The point of this whole little tale of terror, really, is that what was going on in my workplace was serious, and it threatened my whole professional future. At the time, it felt like the gods were conspiring against me – why else would such madness persist? You had to ask yourself at least that, when things go wrong in life. What had I done to deserve this? How could I make it better?

Aware of how shaky I felt through this ordeal, I had chosen caution, and conversation, and sought a face-to-face meeting to diffuse things (as the university grievance mediation guidelines recommended), hoping for some kind of verbal reassurance. I had agreed to external mediation, even after the findings against my accuser had been passed down, in an effort to reconcile her, and to create goodwill, to be a good 'academic citizen': our graduate students not to mention the staff were all affected by this dispute. Surely, I thought, we can talk: this is Australia. This is Lismore. I grew up here, for God's sake; this is where I went to high school. North Coast alternative lifestyle discourse (which had defined this part of Australia since the 1970s) had not changed, had it? It was more sophisticated, but it remained one of live-and-let-live, whilst opposing harm. I trusted that good would prevail. A whole adult life lived in London and moving in privileged professional worlds had further reassured me of this, at least – that it was the proper thing, the Australian thing, indeed the only decent thing to do, to be a team player, to keep things close, to not make a fuss, to not give air to a fire that no one wanted be warmed by. And there it was, that big, fat, American-style letter: welcome to the Rainbow Region, 21st century style. Keep your innocent little mouth shut, sweetheart. Bonfire thick, it was, that letter. Who had talked me into attending that daylong mediation meeting anyway? Who benefitted from the outcome? Not me. Everyone was there protecting their own precious backsides, and there I was, an old hippy sucker, stuck in a time warp, getting bulldozed yet again. I spent most of the day vomiting in the toilets from stress.

At that time, waiting to be called into a meeting to discuss a matter that had, it was rumoured, already cost the university over 50 000 dollars in legal fees, I was four months into a nightmare that had seen me on the front page of the national broadsheet education press, accused of plagiarism, with leaked 'papers' reproduced by an 'anonymous' source. The veracity of the papers or indeed the legitimacy of the claim had never been verified by the journalist: no one had bothered to contact me. Through all this, I had not missed one single day of work. I had not cried off a single lecture, or tutorial, or staff meeting, or any obligation and duty, despite the horror of having to face a crowd of students that, like any small community, had their singular attachments to scandal and gossip. And I continued to work side by side with staff that had betrayed me, and helped my accuser prosper in her bankrupt campaign. Frankly, the whole faculty had known about it for some time, and no one had even had the human decency to pull me aside and warn me. Only two members of staff ever apologised to me for their conduct. They remain the only two people I trust amongst all my academic colleagues from that institution.

I thought that my behaviour throughout the whole affair had been exemplary. But who knows? Certainly, I neglected my children. Certainly, I should not have written such forthright comments on my accuser's draft PhD (its standard had shocked me); perhaps, being so readily shocked, I revealed myself as a cultural misfit within the institution; perhaps I should have stuck gold stars all over her manuscript, tried that kind of exemplary behaviour instead; then none of this would have happened. Perhaps. Then again, it might have been an accident waiting to happen, any time, anywhere, and the small details of character and place were, in reality, utterly insignificant. But then, I had no such philosophy intact, and my patience was worn out. Many of my colleagues did not speak to me. Graduate students ditto. The woman in question continued to harass me. I duly complained. I duly waited for a suitable reaction. None came. Until that big thick fat letter, and now, this meeting. Please, I prayed: let this end.

These are some things that I knew to be true. I wasn't a plagiarist. I had written more books, published more academic articles, than anyone else in the whole faculty, save the dean. Still, that was the sound echoing in my horrified head: *shut up shut up shut up you big fat moaner. Laugh it off. Go surfing. Shut up. Stop protesting, stop professing your talents.* I wish I had. But no: instead of trusting my intuition, which had me feeling squalid, I turned not on my accuser, but on the people that were meant to be managing her, and me. I was not responsible for what she had done, or what they had done to her in their handling of the matter, were still doing, but it was also happening to me and I wanted it to stop. The other truth was harder to acknowledge. I had given up so much of my life for this career, at first, to establish myself, and later, simply to protect my family. In doing so, I had neglected them. To my shame, I have a photo of me breastfeeding my first-born baby, typing on a laptop at the same time, trying to meet a publishing deadline, which if met would result in a published book and land me an academic job. It did – was it worth it? – well, I guess that's why I'm writing this book, to take account. This pattern never stopped. Weaning babies to go to work to earn a living because your husband is unemployed. Working most weekends marking essays. Disappearing for long absences for research and conferences. It is true, I was guilty of putting the demands of publishers first, but only because I thought this would allow me to keep my (contracted) positions, allow me in turn to then face the needs of my babies. If I had this equation wrong, I would pay for it forever, but did I have to let what was happening right here and now be the deciding factor? Was it fair that all that sacrifice should come down to this – to someone saying that I 'stole' other people's words, and for the telling of that lie and the management of the scandal surrounding it to undo me forever? Please not.

I announced myself to the VC's secretary. Unable to take a seat, I almost left. I imagined myself turning the key in the car, driving away from this valley, down to the sea, and packing. Flying back to London. I could almost feel the grinding joy that is Terminal 3 at Heathrow. The long-but-much-loved bus ride (now no longer in service) back into London proper. Turning the key of our front door, our empty house, tripping gently against the empty milk bottles. Back from a good day's teaching, and in between bursts of writing, gazing from my office in the university across the Thames to St Paul's Cathedral. Our nanny smiling with freshly washed babies in her arms. Friends due for supper. Stories to be read. Wine to be opened. That once-upon-a-time reality was now a long-lost fantasy.

'You can come in now', the secretary announced. Clearly, this was my reality. Here, now, I was about to pick a fight with my acting vice chancellor. I was mad as hell. I was hell's menopausal divorcée with a hangover. How mad, I did not at the time fully understand. Like poor Ophelia, 'Divided from herself and her fair judgement', I had no idea how far from fullness or rationality I in fact was.

Thirty-five minutes later I was back in my office. There had been some screaming. It had not been pleasant. It had all come out of my mouth. It had been directed at two poor, weak, gutless men who were only my enemies because they were not my defenders – who can afford to be ethical and principled in the 21st century? They did probably not deserve my wrath (though one of them, it disgusts me to relate, had a fondness for public displays of loosely elasticised G-strings at staff Christmas parties), but there we all unfortunately were, in the same office, unwilling players in an unwinnable game of three-handed political poker. There had been flooding humiliations of tears that had been damming up for months (from me). I had not stopped crying. All this in response to the simple opening claim that I had been well supported. I had managed to be divorced, had been through more property settlements than your average 40-year-old, written too many (regrettably) published poems about lost love and kingdoms of idealised parenthood to think that something as trivial as *work* could rank as a life-scuttling force. *I am going home to surf. And be quiet. Be. Quiet.* Twenty-six students a year in Australian Literature at the University of London and that was worthy of the prime minister's congratulations, yet now I have to manage over 300 each semester plus postgraduates and I don't know all their names and *have you read our kindly reminder letter telling you how very lucky you are to have a job at this prestigious institution*, soon to celebrate its 10th birthday? *Shame on you.*

'The university has fully supported you', they said. I did not feel supported. We have done nothing wrong, they said next. I felt skewered. I could tell they were frightened, but not as frightened as I was. At that time, I did not appreciate what the men in that room had to lose by siding with me. Now, I feel that I have served a cold-fired apprenticeship for poker-faced management, watching their mastery in handling me. I can, now, retrospectively understand that in a conflict between two 'unstable, volatile' staff members, particularly if the staff members are women, I too would be mightily pleased for such matters to be dealt with by my 'Acting'. In prisons, human beings are raped by their fellow human beings: violence is magnified in institutional settings. Outside prison, we like to believe in the exercise of free will, and try to believe that we will never become a statistic of violence. How well do we all behave? Honestly? Why is it that large institutions, like universities, are so prone to withdrawal from reasonable human conduct, so often hothouses for psychopaths, so bad at being held to account that they must routinely offer up innocents as collateral damage? And there I was, believing that I had written my PhD to enter a vocation devoted to higher things. The university as a (failing) factory sector is not something I understood enough to protect myself from.

Needless to say, the meeting ended badly. I was shaking uncontrollably, and sobbing as though another character had inhabited my grief: the sounds were not recognisably mine. I was dismissed. I was asked to leave the room. No one offered me any kind of help; the administrative staff averted their eyes. I walked back to my office, with people staring at me everywhere, thinking of how much credit I had available on my cards, to facilitate a dramatic leave-taking for good. Two of my concerned colleagues, whom I was due to meet with regarding course development, were waiting in my office, and watched me neatly organise my work into varying piles of responsibilities to delegate, write a brief note of instruction to the mythical person who was (never) to replace me, then walk out of the door and back down that ramp to the car park for what I truly believed would be the last time. I was gone.

Half a year later in calendar terms – but galaxies away if measuring experiential worlds – I was back at work. In the intervening period, because I had been designated as having suffered a psychological injury at work, I visited more doctors, psychologists, and psychiatrists than imaginable, and all of it was compulsory – if I wanted my pay cheque to continue, that is. I continued to see my last psychiatrist, the only one that really helped me, on a voluntary basis until I moved to Melbourne some years later. It was he who understood and unpacked the long history of me, in particular, the torture of depression that had been haunting me since becoming a mother. To say that he diagnosed me with postnatal depression would be as useless as describing day as being the opposite of night, and would belittle the true diagnostic artistry that is involved when one human being defines another. He gave me a language to describe and understand the pain of selfhood, aka me. But, in July 2004, I knew nothing except that I was falling, and I had no desire to save myself.

That was then, and this is now, as they say. What do we do when things go wrong in life? I suspect that we don't really know what we do, that we'd be much better at describing how other people around us react to adversity. I had an aunty who used to start humming and clicking her tongue. She was a nurse, who married for the first but not the last time in her seventies. I know people who talk a lot of nervous nonsense, and often it is entertaining. People who pick fights. And entire platoons of people who fit into the 'fright and flight' category. What I think about me is this: when I am at my most threatened, my desire to please and appease goes into overdrive. I am not by nature (or should I say nurture?) a 'fuck you' person, but rather a 'please don't fuck with me' person. So what had happened back there in that office was a world first for me, and it felt like the end of something. Perhaps even me. I don't remember the long drive home. I don't remember phoning and making an appointment to see my doctor. I seemed to emerge into a different consciousness a few days later. Recalling that my doctor had signed me off work, I had the wits to post but not the manners to explain the bunch of paperwork I confusedly sent off to the director of human resources. I thought, 'I'll be OK next week', but it was more than half a year before I walked up that wooden ramp to the Arts Faculty again.

What *do* we do when things go wrong? A pear-shaped life appears to be the new ergonomic cradle for more and more people these days. Can we learn anything from adversity, truly? As I lay down in the cradle of my own adversity back then, I rocked, and did not get up for a very long time, and it seemed there was nothing around, like a map, to help me navigate myself away from pain. I thought that is what therapy was meant to provide, cartography for salvation. Well, for the most part therapy failed me and I failed it, which is another reason why I determined to write this book.

Have I moved far enough away from pain to make sense? It remains to be seen, and perhaps you, dear reader, will be the judge of whether or not wisdom is the true bridegroom of my experience. Every single book or memoir of postnatal depression that I have read advocates the beatific advice of therapy. There is a recognisable pattern to all of the narratives I read – denial, breakdown, confession of need for help, an account of the benefits of medical and therapeutic intervention and their salvations, and the glory of recovery. My own story was not that shapely, or linear, or redemptive. And that is enough of a reason to share my mess – if you have postnatal depression or know people who do, if you have ever wished a baby away and feel that the grip of that grief will never leave, then this messy narrative is for you. Depression for me felt like a cruel origami from hell, and in this narrative I am trying, still, to unfold myself so that you can see my pretty paper, with all its creases. The imprint of the shape I once was will always be visible.

Once you enter the world of the 'categorised' mentally ill, it is forever your world, even when well. One of the most curious aspects about this belief for me – maybe it is the historian in me – is defining when it began. This question still preoccupies me. People around you, with or without permission, can be surprisingly forthcoming with their own views on the subject. If you can manage to keep a sense of humour about it, these 'historic' readings of 'you as the subject; topic: madness' can be outrageously entertaining, even if to suggest that perspectives on the past are so sinewed with individuality that I am amazed consensus has ever been a societal possibility. I feel a little stupid that I had believed people thought of me as a hard-working, solid, loyal, friendly, polite, and a fun person, if a little bossy, and that this belief turned out to be largely inaccurate. The bossy bit seemed spot on (I have always been perfectly capable of disliking myself, but never training myself out of less than congenial behaviours). As my 1969 kindergarten report read, 'Susan is very popular but she likes to organise the other children into lines'. How embarrassing. Stupid. People – so I found out as they told me for the first time after having my nervous breakdown (I need to repeat that, *my nervous breakdown*) – had quite a different idea of me, or additional ideas. They thought me secretive. Private. Loopy. Loud. Scatterbrained. Stubborn. Inflexible. Argumentative. Some more complimentary appraisals had me down as generous (to the point of idiocy), irresponsibly irrepressible, and hugely energetic and inspirational (with the downside that this made people feel inferior). I thought two things at once as this was all revealed to me. Not only did people not know who I really was, but possibly nor did I. Would I ever escape my kindergarten self?

Was all this my fault? Who am I? I held this dilemma close, but when I was at my most ill, I did not have the energy for the resourceful consideration such a dilemma required. I still don't. And though it saddens me, for the present I concentrate all my efforts in trying to ensure that no such falsehoods exist within my immediate family; that I keep the barriers down. It is an endless chore and I wonder if I will ever properly achieve it. But I must keep trying because otherwise I will never begin to understand what happened. And despite every Tom, Dick and Harriet having their own opinions about the origins of my weird self, for this story the only two narratives that matter are mine and the medical ones. They overlap in that double helix kind of way. But it is quite sobering how far apart they can be from each other, these narratives, which can be very disturbing in a quest for truth.

Anyone who has been diagnosed with a mental illness or knows people who have been (or perhaps think they should be!) will recognise part of this story. Part of the story that I am keen to document, however, is how the process of being diagnosed and cared for – particularly if you are an employee, and if insurance payments are involved in covering your wages – involves endless testing that in my opinion was insulting and harmful. Driving hours and hours to Brisbane in resentful tropical downpours to see the insurer's psychiatrist when you yourself are as mad as a cyclone is not really my idea of road safety. Or a good time. I had to tell the story of how I got so depressed to so many different kinds of people, so many times that I felt myself belonging to the medical military: specimen woman; mad version. Abusive story: clumsy, irresponsible employer at fault therefore they must pay.

Reading the medical reports later, they all acknowledged that I had had recent and significant stress in my life prior to the psychological injury that had occurred at work. Some even diagnosed post-traumatic stress syndrome related to Scarlet's near death in London, and severe postnatal depression, but they all agreed about one thing: that it was the workplace injury that was responsible for my current condition, and that my condition was being exacerbated by the lack of closure (to be precise, my complaint not being processed). Oh yes, that was another thing that my friends and family revealed, that I had completely, insanely, unrealistic expectations of people and institutions. I was always more angry at the university than my accuser, because I felt they had a greater responsibility, but now I hope I am wiser. What would *I* have done if *I* were VC? Who knows what generals go through to make their decisions? Or mothers that can choose only one child to save. My situation was and is small, small bikkies comparatively, and I am forever shamed to have been undone by such a tiny, dismal thing as falling over and not being able to get up simply because someone was not playing by my moral rules. Yes, they are right, I am inflexible, and hope not to be anymore. It can be extremely bad for one's health. One thing I will tell you though is this: while I was falling and fallen, the view from below may have been ugly, but it was as revealing as skates on fresh ice. I saw the precise nature of the ugliness of many of the people with whom I continued to have to work side by side, practising but failing miserably to grasp forgiveness. Work should not be like that.

Like I imagine there are in true combat zones, there were also angels. A principled, ethical person is a rare thing. If they are also astute, then you are blessed to have them on your side. There was one such dean at my university. I remember him picking me up off the floor outside the room where the investigating committee had interviewed me after I had collapsed. Telling me it would be all right. That he'd sort them out. That he had heard what I'd said. He had asked me then, away from formal scrutinising, why I thought she'd done it. I told him I thought it was jealousy. Horizontal hostility amongst women is vicious. I also said I thought she was a bit crazy, possibly because of her own health problems which had her examining death earlier than anyone would want to. I said that she had not spoken to me since I returned her thesis with my comments. I said that beyond this I had no idea other than that she clearly didn't like me. I said I thought my department had not done a particularly good job of postgraduate leadership, and I had not done a particularly good job of being sensitive about these failings. He made a good diagnosis, about my integrity, and he went into those laborious meetings and spoke on my behalf. But it was a long time before I felt the victory of his trust, his diagnosis. A diagnosis takes talent to make. To assert it, takes more courage than most of us possess.

When Scarlet was in a coma at Great Ormond Street Hospital for Children in London, when she was 9 months old, at that time when the long decision to leave London had begun, they were all like that, those doctors in paediatric intensive care. World-class diagnosticians. Different medical teams were fighting over her, adrenalin-fuelled, trying to 'win' a diagnosis. What had happened? The team that got it – metabolics – was the quietest. They asked the best questions, and listened to our story, feeling the clues surface like clots. They saved her life. My children were the only two children in the UK to have that particular mutation of the MCADD genes. I'll tell you properly about MCADD when this story catches up to itself, when I talk about Scarlet's birth. But for now, it is enough to know that when they get ill, they are the only kids in Australia to get ill in the way they do. They are medical mysteries, or novelties, living research subjects with a condition that is less than two decades from point of discovery.

Scarlet and Hunter have MCADD, but James and I gave it to them, because it is genetically inherited. One of the most humiliating things about having sick children is how unsaintly the experience can be at times, and how ungracious an exhausted parent's behaviour can become. We all of us inhabit human bodies, and are too often self-centred. When Scarlet was in her coma, the one that led to her lifelong diagnosis, James and I were dashing off still to vomit, and fight off whatever illness it was that had brought the whole family to its knees. We could not eat even if we wanted to, so we were in a most diminished capacity when it comes to being fit to cope and deal with a normal situation let alone this one. But I also mean something else when I say the kids have the MCADD but we, *we* – oh yes, what about us? We have to manage it. We have to cope. I cannot enter a hospital now without vomiting from panic. James has to go, mostly, initially, until I muster my performative self. Divide and rule. But sometime, sometimes, I have gone. And on the day that I went, when Scarlet had her first ambulance ride in Australia, that was the day of straw and concrete.

EXISTENTIAL EQUATIONS, MAD TESTS

This, this was when I fell over, when the pear became an unrecognisable fruit, a suddenly poisonous one. And because I had never let myself feel what had happened to Scarlet, properly, at any time, because of absolute petrified fear, because this refusal to feel was sinful, I truly believed that I was being punished. I believed I deserved it, but I did not know why. That was what I had to find out: why was this thing happening to me, in this way, in this place, at this time? When I did this, found out these answers, then no one could hurt my children anymore. It was as if I believed that the very worst thing had to happen to me in the exact combination that it did, and that this was a challenge presented to me: it was my final chance to get it right, otherwise one of my children was going to die.

These were my first thoughts when I read that email from my postgrad student asking me if I was a plagiarist. It was like a near death experience, with the future bedlam yet to come flashing before me, preview style. Everything I feared was embedded in that accusation: it was not the falsehood of outing me as a plagiarist that was my concern; the real terror was my fraudulent claim to motherhood. That is where I was a great pretender. I was not a good mother, I was not a real mother, I did not deserve to name myself a mother. I was masquerading as something I was not, and I was vulnerable to exposure. I had children, sure, but would they give me a motherhood licence if there was such a test? I hardly thought so. Small wonder that when accused of something I absolutely was not, I fought tooth and nail to defend my honour, lest the truth seekers snuck in the back and found out my true secret. Then they would take Scarlet away from me, because I was an imposter. And I was not going to allow that.

Clearly, written down, or spoken aloud, this narrative qualifies me immediately for the madhouse, on the one hand. But on the other, how many of us are really rational all the time? How many of us don't walk under ladders or avoid treading on cracks, laughing at ourselves at the same time, but all the same wary of the possible consequences of courting disaster? Madness might be nothing more than superstition writ large. I believed, almost instantaneously, that this challenge had been set as a test: if I could survive this, then nothing would ever hurt Scarlet again. If I did not, if my enemies defeated me, then I was unworthy of being a mother. That's right, isn't it?

TO BE OF GOOD HEART

'Life is certainly not without its challenges for you . . .' and 'Given the difficulties of your lives at present . . .', write our friends in their notes to us. I love the manners of the English, and may god bless every stationery supplier in the nation, and the posties, and all the lovely notes that are now fond memories and curios for future generations. But I am shocked to read, looking at them these few years later, of the concern and distress that people close to us were expressing: 'I can hardly believe you have the time to buy a loaf of bread, let alone . . .' the normal things that define functioning, social human behaviour, like buying baby gifts, or remembering the birthdays of those people you love or respect.

But one of my favourite letters from a steadfast friend ends, after acknowledging the chaos of our life, and offering a spare room whenever we needed (as they lived around the corner from GOSH), 'In the meantime, be of good heart, lots of love . . .' One must: be of good heart. When things go pear shaped, and your mind takes a chemical holiday from normality, and the train never arrives on time, to be of good heart is a grace worth praying for. And it is something that can indeed be cultivated. I sometimes go to church to do this, often for no other reason than to be reminded that the ego is something worth rendering as less important than we constantly believe it to be. That human suffering is widespread, historical, and not without context.

Ask this of the disease depression: 'What do you look like, smell like, why did you come here, what do you want, what lessons are you teaching the world?' Whatever it is that illness can teach us, I believe that lesson to be the real truth of disease, (and for disease, insert 'all that can go wrong in life'). And I believe that the only lesson worth learning is the one of grace. When I have space in me that allows health to return to full occupancy, when I am peaceful and functioning, which is often, it is then that I can most afford to train my heart up for goodness, and I do. I fail daily. I am surprised, for example, that my husband has not left me, that my children still seem to love me, and that I have any friends remaining that actually seek me out. I fail big time. But, I must also win some. And if I didn't ask of my mental condition, 'What are you teaching me?' or if I didn't interrogate MCADD as a medical condition (literally, metaphorically, through writing) to locate its finer value, if I did not as a writer continually explore the true shape of pears, then I would be my own worst enemy: simply someone, of no good heart.

But, there are times when it has been different.

Chapter 2

My first babies, and the historical claws of illness

The most beautiful moment in my life was when the man I loved said he wanted to make babies with me. 'I love you', and 'Will you marry me' don't come anywhere close as statements that shook my world. Once, a woman of my mother's generation said to me, remarking on my numerous marriages/partnerships, and despite the fact that she had herself been married for decades, that she would have given anything to have been romantically wooed, to have felt that she was 'the chosen one'. 'You don't know how lucky you are for someone to ask you to marry you', she said to me. 'I was pregnant, and it was just a miserable decision we had to go through with'. After a sad pause, she concluded, 'my whole life felt like the consequence of an accident. He would never have married me otherwise'.

It is true that this was not my experience – both my husbands surprised me with their marriage proposals, and I had been asked by three other men that I'd had meaningful relationships with (and another scoundrel who was very cute but just wanted an Australian passport). But certainly, my early pregnancies which were aborted (and that sentence alone is the hardest one I have written in this book) and the two pregnancies in my first marriage, were unplanned. But the experience was a long way away indeed from the 'shotgun wedding' scenario so many live with.

The first question that my first midwife asked was 'Is this a planned pregnancy?' When I answered no, worried that this would make me seem somehow irresponsible and undesiring of the baby, she said that only about 10% were, in her experience. What an alarming statistic, when you think about it, that such major life change for so many in society is begun from that premise, from that less-than-sure place. Surely this must contribute to the prevalence of postnatal depression? The experience in my second marriage to James, which resulted in Scarlet and Hunter's birth, was interplanetary in its difference. When a man asks you to be the mother of his children, then takes you to bed to work on that project, it brings not only a new physical but, also, for me, spiritual dimension to lovemaking that I had never before experienced. And now that that time in my life is over, nothing, *nothing* makes me feel older. So yes, to have been 'chosen' in that way was a life-altering experience, and such a strong and beautiful one that without it as a living memory, I doubt I would have survived my postnatal depression in the way I did. You never can tell what might have otherwise happened, but when I most felt like surrendering, it was the knowledge that I had chosen this path, hand in hand with my husband, and that it was once the most beautiful decision imaginable – well, that can unplug a constipated heart.

This chapter is about all my pregnancies, and the circumstances surrounding them, and their lived consequences. One thing I definitely did not know when I was younger – an adult, nevertheless – was that the things you decide and do remain with you forever. Alive and kicking. Memories pack punches. Every man I have ever kissed is part of my emotional DNA, and I can't undo any of it, as much as I might like to rewrite history. I truly believe that this is where postnatal depression began for me, in all that reckless kissing and sex and procreation and killing. If there is one truth I would like my children to know it would be this: your decisions stay with you for life, and you can feel their echo forever. Kissing is no frivolous business. My personal history of kissing has a lot to answer for. Those answers are part of the story of my own understanding of postnatal depression, and recovery.

Telling the truth about the past involves recognising that your life might not have turned out to be how you thought it would, or should. When you admit this, you also have to acknowledge the things that have gone wrong, the things that have got in the way of you and your imagined life, and examine them. Attending this examination, for me, was a great sense of mourning. It is right to grieve for the things we have lost, but grief is not always on its best behaviour when you are as depressed as a wet bucket of sand. Guilt played an overlarge part in the opera of grief that accompanied examining my miscarriage, and divorce, and subsequent pregnancies. Was it because of my earlier, lackadaisical attitudes towards abortion and fertility? Had I taken love for granted? Did I wish my baby away? Were my two youngest children born with a major, life-threatening condition because it was wrong to choose a love that resulted in two other young children being rendered fatherless, and another with a 'substitute'? Divorce and remarriage – who can ever figure out the true costs?

Guilt. Good grief. That topic is worth exploring, because it was a monumentally vital factor in my depression. Some mornings, off to yoga I trotted for a 6am class, abandoning the children to a father who was often unable to speak for two hours, so stunned was he by these early mornings and their foreign demands. There I would sit, listening to the tide shifting on nearby Seven Mile Beach (don't you love the way Australians name beaches so inventively after mileage?), concentrating on healing. I tried so hard to urge my body to wellness, but I felt so guilty, mostly about being sick, but about everything, actually. This list included leaving London, leaving our home and its safety, taking my husband away from his children from his first marriage, stopping breastfeeding, failing at work – the list was endless. Guilt, that demon that frustrates our desires. Then I'd go home, a few hours later, to a combustible place, where guilt was the kindling wood about to burn my life down. Being sick, and thinking about the past, and trying to reassert your needs when your life has collapsed: it is not easy.

One day, I chanted to myself, one day, guilt will fly away. Be prepared for what might come: I was good at being prepared, or so I thought. Mind you, the benefits of a yoga session are rapidly undone by re-entering the madhouse that 8am in a family of five can be. My poor neighbours, I would always think, as I neared home. What must they think of me? Why were the kids always screaming? Why wasn't I coping with this better? *Make babies with me. Make babies with me.*

Any expert will tell you that pregnancy can be a tricky period for women in terms of the past haunting you with its sad little waltz through what should be a genuinely happy time. But pregnancy is also traditionally a time when you come to terms with things, in a psychological sense, almost like spring-cleaning the soul. For me, the first pregnancy that I carried to term therefore involved being confronted with many things that I had not given due consideration to. These ranged from a strong history of sexual misdemeanour, to the psychological and physical rejection of both my homeland and family, and the more existential dilemma of 'what am I really meant to be doing with my life?'

I will never forget the look on the midwife's face in antenatal classes, when, week after week, in answer to all her very real questions about very real scenarios – *and what will you do when the baby cries for the tenth time in the night?* – I said 'let the nanny deal with it'. I recognise her look, now, from this long distance, as one of great concern. She probably clocked that I was in some kind of denial. How I wish she had spoken to me, or sought me out privately. Perhaps I was an unlikeable student. But that was me: pregnant, and more focused on securing a job as soon as the baby was born, and employing the right 'help', than imagining anything about motherhood other than it being something that must be managed. After all, nothing had come between me and my life before – why start now? Have I mentioned shame yet?

The first time I was pregnant, as an undergraduate at university in Sydney, engaged to a prominent rock musician (don't ask – and I was doomed to repeat this tragedy) it was a surreal experience. First, factually, not many people at that time in Australia went to university. Second, no one my age, in my 'inner-city-rock' scene bothered with 'engagements', so we were odd and eccentric in embracing this act of commitment, in our circle, at least. Third, not only was I at university, I was working as a rock journalist, a woman in a then largely male domain of music journalism, and to make matters more complicated I was also a well-known, loud-mouthed, dedicated, protest-marching feminist (and co-author of our radical university newspaper, where I routinely aired these views). What a bifurcated life I led. I was that sad kind of feminist, the kind who would cook a huge meal for the entire band and proceed to lecture them about women's oppression whilst they drank all the beer I had, naturally, paid for. After hours of rock gigs it was not unthinkable to seek out girlfriends at local lesbian haunts. Go figure. Perhaps the most feminist thing about me at this time was that, as a result of having just researched and published an article on contraception and women's health, I knew the best abortion clinic in Sydney.

'Best' from my point of view was a clinic run by a feminist collective in the harbourside suburb of Balmain. 'Best' was a clinic that did not have a posse of 24/7 'pro-life' protesters crowding the footpath like at my local clinic in Surry Hills. 'Best'. Wow, what a concept. How does a young girl, which is what I consider my own students of the same age to be despite the fact that they are living independent lives at university, how does this young girl decide what 'best' is? Like hundreds of other girls that week, I had to make that decision on my own. I was estranged from my family (my mother had run off with a man younger than my little brother, flitting off to far north Queensland, as you do, and my father was a drunken mess, who had sabotaged all my attempts to get myself to university so he was hardly approachable about my consequent mess) and my fiancé was at rehearsals for an imminent recording. Studio time costs a lot of money; my abortion did not seem significant in comparison. So. I travelled on public transport for an hour and a bit over to the clinic in the early morning, and splurged on the complete luxury of a taxi home in the late afternoon – by which time my fiancé (of not too much longer, it has to be said) was back from 'work' with some celebratory beer under his arm. To cheer me up. How thoughtful. I drank with him, and then vomited.

Maybe the saddest thing about this day was that I discovered by sheer accident some months later that one of my housemates had had an abortion on that very same day, at that very same clinic. We did not move in completely the same circles, but we shared a home, shopped together, and cooked together. We were from the same country town. I only found out because I caught her unawares, crying, on the stairs, over some lover's cruelty. She was not normally one for chummy, girly confessions, but she knew that I had known this man, her man, since high school. They had been together a long time, and that was the first and only time I heard her slander him (and, they are still together, a quarter of a century later). But on that day, she was thinking about leaving. The fight was over a small, inconsequential thing, so it turned out, but her 'is he worth it, should I leave him' lament came from the same place that my anguish resided: you can never take it back, what you leave behind in an abortion clinic. And if you've never had to endure the abortionist's final internal examination determining the age of the foetus, just before the local anaesthetic is administered (this I forever regret – I wish I had opted for the general) then you can never truly feel the decision to end a life. It is women's business. And, largely, women's pain.

I say this, but – there are men who seem to have never recovered from the experience either. Perhaps 'recovered' is the wrong word, implying as it does that everything ungainly, unsightly, and unpleasant has been reupholstered to a shiny 'as new' brilliance. Where do our proper and rightful memories reside, in such a process? Are they the old stuffing in the renovated cushion, squashed and suffocated in a modern corset? And what is the alternative? Embroidering the names or shape of our dead babies on your best party frock for all to see? Recently, my husband James came home from a research trip to the UK, and his funny, cute little gift for me was a key ring, with a reproduction of the startling beautiful red and white British wartime poster with the symbol of the crown and the stiff advice to 'Keep Calm and Carry On'. In my culture, that is what we do. Is that a brown snake over there? Well get a bloody shovel and deal with it and get on with what you are meant to be doing. The men go to the pub and the women have their own sly worlds and the children are Victorian in their independent forbearance, and so on and so on and so on, harvest after harvest after season after season, war after war. We all carry on. Some of us collapse, but there is always the knowledge that in some cultures it is right and proper to be left to die in such circumstances.

Do women really own the pain of loss? Yes, we own the memory, of the physical gore of abortion or miscarriage, but not necessarily the psychological trauma that accompanies this. The well-known Australian writer Peter Carey has written about his own experience of abortion, and the grief that he harbours long after the event. It was published in one of those weekend colour supplements that come with your Saturday papers, and I remember the shock of reading it – it seemed so out of character, this confessional tone, from such a familiar voice. It was 1994, a few years before my eldest daughter was born, and a decade after my own visit to that Balmain clinic. I was sitting at a café across the road from Bronte Beach in Sydney, reading, then embarrassing my poor (first) husband Matthias with my blubbering. *What's wrong honey?* How can you sensibly answer that question? Ever since that Balmain morning, I have an imaginary daughter. She is 27 years old now. She has lived a big life.

I was wearing a yellow cotton Indian dress the day my GP told me I was pregnant, and shortly afterwards handed me the contact details for a local abortion clinic. She had been judgemental and unkind, and when I walked outside into the muggy sunshine, dazed, anybody would be a welcome sight after the look in her eyes. My breasts ached. My fiancée was sitting in a bus shelter, avoiding the heat. How are you going to get rid of it, he asked. We went to the beach. A few weeks later, I had an abortion. I never see that man now – but I wonder, what does he feel? Nothing probably. Taking his emotional temperature is not that difficult, if one can trust journalism: in a recent interview (him being still quasi-famous) he was quoted as declaring marriage to be 'a pointless religious exercise' – (What? Getting married was his idea! People still talk about our engagement party – and not just because I went home with the guitarist in another band, *see I told you so, kissing is dangerous*) – and that 'overpopulation is the cause of everything bad'. That's fine. He's fine. Guilt-free and pain-free. For me, things are different, and getting worse. I have my imaginary daughter; she might phone me up later and let me know how she's doing.

There was another catastrophic misdemeanour of this same kind not so long afterwards. I became pregnant by 'the guitarist' (a world-class womaniser after his true love had spurned him) and had to suffer another abortion. After I found out I was pregnant, he climbed up a tree onto my balcony one night very late (knowing that my fiancé was on tour, but politely avoiding my housemates nonetheless) and burst into my room like a revolutionary prowler. Unfortunately, his visit was too late as sadly I had 'fixed' things already. But he at least had the humanity to care about what had passed. I remember us both feeling sad, and chastened. He is a solid and devoted family man now, by all accounts. I saw him last summer (he is still famous) at a reunion gig, with his son now in the band. That sure messed with my head. I spent a large part of the evening listening to music that was decades old in a room with people who were really far too aged to be shaking their bodies around like they were, thinking about what might have been. Unseemly acts. We never loved each other singularly, but we were always steadfast friends in a way that only kids from the country were in that scene, and had been lovers on and off for years. The mess we had got ourselves into with an unwanted pregnancy made us both miserable, but with the aplomb of the young we just kept on living our glorious lives. The guitarist went off on his international tour; my fiancé came back, and we promptly split up. A quarter of a century later, backstage smells the same as it always has. I introduced the guitarist to a husband of mine he hadn't met – the last time we'd seen each other I was pregnant with Ulrike and he bought me a book about baby massage, telling me to do it every night, warning me not to miss this precious thing in life. It was all so, so long ago, but so, so sad. Unspeakably sad – you just don't bring those things up in normal conversation. It was 3am, late in 2009, too late for regrets.

But I sincerely regret not having our child. What can you do with such regret? We shared a cigarette – even that is illegal now – on the footpath outside the venue, while the band truck was being loaded. It was 2am. I don't smoke. His son is a wonderful young man. How did we make those decisions of so long ago? Where did we get the courage? Do we ever really forget?

For Peter Carey, it was a different matter entirely, dealing with his past decisions. His essay article, 'My lasting wish' is a sad lament for his lost/aborted/miscarried children. He writes about thinking about his children, not just the ones who are alive, and waiting to be taken to sport, but his dead babies. His wish is that he had honoured their passing in a more fitting way. Writing such a moving story serves as an act of honour, you could say. His pain was not an unfamiliar one, just one not routinely discussed, certainly not in major broadsheets of the time. Alan Close, another Australian writer famed for his concern with men's issues, and a long-time friend of mine, has also publicly related his experiences of lost fatherhood, calling himself 'the father of several terminations'. Like others, he imagines his child at the age 'he' might otherwise have been. But, instead of parenting, he described this dormant love as 'hardening in my bones'. Despite his dream of becoming a father later being realised, Alan reminds us that long after the event, women and men both grieve the loss of an unborn child.

Post-abortion syndrome is a disorder that I had never heard of, but one which makes sense to me now, as I look back on the grief that contributed to the demise of my first marriage, and most certainly to my subsequent postnatal depression. It is interesting that Peter and Alan's stories testify to this practice of 'carrying on', which we all do too much of, and how this in turn creates a new category of regret. If we deny the real pain of what happened, *have another beer, Susie* then 'surprise surprise' if this denial does not come back to bite us in the bottom one day – for me, it was there each time I became pregnant, and had to pay due attention to the imaginary life of my lost family, the babies I had killed.

BECOMING A MOTHER

I was dearly in love with my first husband, Matthias, when we fell pregnant with our eldest daughter, Ulrike. I was in my early thirties, and we had already been married for 10 years at that time. She has just started high school as I write this, and is already taller than me. Of all the memories created between then and now, it is incredible that I can recall so horribly the postnatal depression – why should it have such precedence after all this time? I want to write it away. More, I wish I could have the time all over again.

It was mid winter of 1996, in London, and I had just been shopping. My new overcoat was nothing short of fabulous. Having grown up in the Australian subtropics, winter clothes had not been a large part of my life, so this was a distinct bonus about living in London – the endless opportunities to layer yourself in cashmere and wrap yourself in mighty, woollen overcoats. We lived in a garden flat in Fulham in the Royal Borough of Kensington and Chelsea, in a long, thin street running off the North End Road where the street markets did an impressive trade. Here you could buy anything from fruit and vegetables to high-end fashion, all sold off at gritty, street prices. This is where I found it, my long-coveted coat. It was almost black-blue, with a collar that allowed the option of a fake fur trim, which felt witty. The cuffs were huge, and it buttoned at the neck with a dramatic wrap effect that required no further buttons, but instead swung in a swashbuckling style. Roomy enough, I hoped, for a growing belly, for it was December and already snowing, and I was pregnant.

You could assume a new personality with such an item of clothing. It required suitably matching shoes – smart boots probably – it demanded professionalism (no more rocking up to school in my sandy poncho or biker jacket) and perhaps even a new haircut – do mothers do bobs? I was intent on transforming myself from motorbike-pillion-passenger-all-adventurous wife flirting with a career in the London education system to . . . what? A writer and a mother in a famous blue coat? That part was too hard. The purchase of this symbol of maturity would have to suffice while plans firmed. I bought some food, and a cute, squat Christmas tree to be collected later, and headed home to contemplate the future, looking a sight in my posh new coat and shod in flip-flops with stripy toe socks. Walking on the early snow in the season of celebration into an unknown future felt fabulous.

When I discovered this pregnancy, and the need to buy a new coat, I had been married for quite a while, but somehow had not really focused on the normal middle-class aspirations to own a home and consolidate your life in a timely manner. Children had never been part of our dreaming. None of our friends had children. We had lived in Germany and Australia, but were married in London's

Wandsworth registry office in March 1988 when we were both in our very early twenties. The marriage certificate recorded 'Courier' and 'Artist' as our occupations. Matthias was a motorcycle courier. It always surprised me how often I would see him racing around the city on his old BMW – what a huge city, what a lot of motorbikes, and there he'd be, streaming down Kensington High Street with awkward shaped parcels, not even noticing me and my mates off down the pub, lunchtime escapees from the art studio for the publishing house where we all worked (I had yet to graduate to the editorial offices). It seemed fitting, somehow, that all these years later our first child was conceived in my favourite place, the city that represented, for me, love, and chance, and freedom. This time around, postgraduate qualifications and PhDs under our belts, we were both working as secondary teachers, believing that we had left Australia for good, and that our little baby was going to be a Londoner. My, how the gods do like to mess with us mortals.

Matthias was as delighted as I had ever seen him when the pregnancy was confirmed, he did not stop smiling for weeks, but then, he panicked. I didn't then, but now, I consider this to be an act of stupidity. Pregnant? No problem. I was offered a job teaching Australian Studies at the University of London. This was a dream-come-true scenario. I told my professor, of course, that I was pregnant. His very sensible response, or so I thought, was, well that's not a problem, teaching doesn't start until October. By all accounts, the baby that we called Lai Lai (Fijian for 'little one') was due in late August. My obstetrician was also excited by my job offer, and offered to induce me three weeks early, so I could 'relax' before starting my new job. It all sounded terribly, terribly sensible.

I was a patient of the Chelsea and Westminster Hospital for this pregnancy, where I attended these antenatal clinics. The waiting rooms were full of classy, rich women, in gorgeous maternity clothes, constantly chattering about outrageously glamorous holiday destinations and their squads of nannies and their impressive and demanding jobs and, most important, when they had 'scheduled' their birth. It seemed abnormal to allow the child to be born on anyone's time plan except yours. So, when my specialists suggested an early C-section, I completely trusted this to be a safe, normal, plan. I agreed.

But Matthias was still worried, and he had a right to be. We had only just begun to establish ourselves in London, and even a month or two on a single income before my return to work would jeopardise our financial well-being. He was lobbying to return to Australia, for an easy life, but also because he was not fond of London any-more. He could not imagine his, or our family's, best life there. His wonderful sister intervened. An academic herself, and archaeologist of note, she knew full well how hard it was to complete postgradu-ate studies successfully, and how it was almost impossible to secure an academic post, let alone such a good one as I had been offered. In a fit of generosity that to this day astounds me, she offered to give us a very large sum of money as a deposit to purchase the flat we were living in, which was coincidentally for sale. For me, it felt like the planets aligning, all this beautiful luck and prosperity and fertility, and the future felt shiny and tremendous. I was in the city I loved best in the world, with my long-time best friends, I was married to a fabulous man whom I loved radiantly, I was soon to have our longed-for baby, and would shortly begin my long-cherished career – all from the base of our own sweet little nest off the Fulham Road.

If I sound like a modern, strong, independent, assertive Western woman, the beneficiary of excellent education and generations of feminist liberation, then this is because I am. It is part of my true chime, but – I am also conservative. I like the man to be the boss. Someone has to be, and I far prefer it not to be me. Matthias said no. He said we were to return to Australia. Not Germany, not London, but Australia. I loved him. I trusted him. Without his concordance, there was only discord in my heart. Before I knew it, we had landed in New York to visit some friends, on our way 'home'. It was fun buying lots of stretchy, funky clothes for my growing belly. It was strange seeing old friends, mostly journalists, and watching them party while I was abstemious. It was fun flying home on an almost empty flight, where we chose our cluster of seats to sleep the journey away in comfort, and enjoyed the rare privilege in economy class of being fed on demand by untaxed air stewards, who kept bringing me special treats for 'the mum and bub'. It was fun coming home to the split-diamond sunshine of Sydney, even if my heart was still in London, and deeply envious that I would not be there to experience the newly elected 'New Labour' government, and the fizz of excite-ment surrounding all that. But, how fabulous, that our daughter would be born in Australia.

Not fun, though, was trying to start a new life, again, and sud-denly having a baby started to feel like quite a frightening thing. We managed, with the help of family and friends. We got ourselves a flat across the road from the beach, a little car, Matthias secured a teaching position and my childhood girlfriend Julie orchestrated a research job for me at her publishing company. Each pay packet we bought things we needed, from washing machines to pushchairs. I swam every day, throughout the winter, and two weeks before my due date I stopped work. Just as well – I had to concentrate better on all the ice cream I needed to eat each day!

I was induced when our baby was two weeks overdue. This was a disappointment, as it meant we could not go to the birthing centre as planned, but in the end I could not have asked for a better birth. Sometimes it was comically tragic – poor Matthias had to conduct a phone interview for a job whilst I was in labour, and Julie shocked and delighted the midwives by bringing in fine china to eat takeaway Thai – but all in all when you compare tales, my first birth experience was a blessed one (am I allowed to moan here about still being able to feel the epidural pain in my back though?) So, what went wrong? How did this happiness turn to suicidal terror?

If I was to write a huge, long list documenting the horrors of my depression and share it with you, I'm not sure what purpose that would achieve. Sure, it would allow women to recognise brands or versions of their own malaise, but that seems like a clinical exercise to me. Because I feel very passionate about this issue, and I do want things to change – is sharing the story enough, without asking some tougher questions? Why wasn't I properly warned? Where was the help when I was desperate? What is wrong with our society that we have trapped ourselves into such a filthy kind of glamour where women are free to work and be their best selves, but lose all that like Scotch mist because our biological bodies have not progressed apace with our aspirations?

Here are some facts about Ulrike's early life and my new life as a mother: Princess Diana was still alive, I had only recently turned down the job for which I had been educating myself for the last 10 years, my husband had two jobs, I had no maternity leave or pay, and not a single one of our friends or close family had children. We had left our fulsome London lives to come home to our imagined paradise, and as a concept it was beginning to feel a little bankrupt. In reality it was just me and a newborn baby, living a stranger's life on the top floor of a beachside flat overlooking the Pacific, which hypnotised me each day. I had lots of visits, which were often stressful as they all expected me to be my normal hostess self, with the exception of three special friends who used to visit and punctuate my loneliness. My writer mate, Al, visited. He had seen Ulrike have her first bath in hospital, and in fact was visiting us in London when I fell pregnant, so he had a spiritual duty to visit, which he fulfilled. He used to swim across Coogee Bay, and come and say hi on his swimming days. Then there was my 'cous' Jen, who usually visited with Julie, a childhood mate from primary school in Coffs Harbour, who had also been at Ulrike's birth. Some nights we watched TV. She did a fabulous line in gourmet takeaway, did Jules, and Jen was the queen of flowers. Thanks to their love and charity, I know what people mean when they describe someone as having a heart of gold. Aside from this, which was not 'nothing', there remained about 90 or so hours of hell each week. Live through this. I lived in the lucky country. The sun did not stop shining. Our flat was modest, but had world-class views and was a cozy home to us. I was not completely alone. But there I was, walking with my baby, chanting *I want my life back*, trying not to fall off the cliff.

Suddenly Matthias lost his job and that was that. Sydney had no rhyme or reason. If it had to be Australia and unemployment, then we were going where everyone went, we were going home to the place with the highest unemployment rate in Australia, we were going to the Far North Coast of New South Wales. We were going home. By Christmas, with Ulrike barely 4 months old, we were there. By the end of the summer break, Matthias and I had both been offered great teaching jobs, him at a school teaching languages by distance and me at the local university in Lismore. Oh, how we pull the archer's bow.

We were living an extended-family life and loving the mundanity of it all, and to top it all had somehow secured the best nanny in the world. Deb had just come back from working in London where she had trained as a nanny. She was a local girl, and had gone to school with some of my cousins. Ulrike loved her instantly. Deb is still the hottest nanny-property in the whole Ballina-Byron shire. When James and I came back to Australia six years later with two more children, and he was spending time with them and a regular at playgroup, he used to sit around and watch the other mothers sigh with envy at Deb's calm, her equilibrium, her talent. She was – is – a Class-A surfie chick, with a special gift. I hope she's not too exhausted from taking care of Lennox Head's bourgeois babies to have her own if that is her dream. She deserves everything.

Back then having Deb in our life probably saved mine. I had no idea I had postnatal depression until I was diagnosed with it years later. I attributed all my unease to the changed circumstances of my life, and constantly chastised myself – be happy, be grateful, be quiet! What did I have to complain about, really? Ulrike was being cared for in an excellent manner, and spending much of her daily life at the beach and playing in the paradise we had chosen. Deb also managed the home exceptionally well, doing domestic chores when Ulrike slept. I came home from work each day to happiness and harmony and a perfectly ordered home. But I was not there. I was emotionally absent. My constant companion was a voice inside my head, walking the long miles of our beautiful beach with me each afternoon with Ulrike in my backpack. Give me my life back, it said. Let me go home to London. Then, around the middle of the year, the job I had turned down in London was advertised again. I applied. I was interviewed by telephone conference by a committee of people I largely did not know and I sat gazing out over the ocean during this lengthy process. Afterwards, they phoned me back almost immediately and offered me the job. I accepted. I was gleeful as a kid at the Royal Easter Show tucking into a showbag full of tantalising treats. Matthias caught my contagious excitement and agreed to go back. What was I doing? I was frightened. I was running away. I was taking flight. I wanted the clay pit of dread that was my constant companion to be gone and this, I thought, was the solution.

We left Australia the day after Ulrike's first birthday. All my chanting had worked. I got my old life back. We arrived in London and slept the divine sleep of the jetlagged for 16 hours in a shabby-chic Bloomsbury B&B, then went to stay with dear friends (Ulrike's godparents, Leonie and Steve) while we waited for our flat to be ready. My work was to begin in a few days. At the time, I thought all my dreams had come true. How I wish I'd known how ill I was in Australia following Ulrike's birth. How I wish that I hadn't hidden it with hard work, with chasing an academic career, with teaching all day and writing yet another book that not enough people would read. But my line of work was a 'publish or perish' one, and not one that necessarily thinks of maternity leave as a legitimate reason for not producing research. Many people might contest this, but at the time I believed only a published book would secure me a tenured academic position. That book, the one that I 'vanished' my depression with, is sitting in the corner of my office right now. In eight, big, recriminating cartons. The publishers kindly sent them to me instead of pulping them. Was it worth it? This question is almost impossible to answer. Yes, that publication and the others that I wrote when I should have been parenting are responsible for my professional success, and definitely helped me win jobs. No, absenting myself in that manner and using work to mask deeper dilemmas was not a good idea. It was a very bad idea. I was deluded. Ill, deluded, and worried about the future. Would I make the same decisions again? No. Never. Will I be able to keep that promise to myself and my children? I hope so. But maybe I need to burn those books instead of letting them stay in the corner of my office, haunting me.

I am mostly interested in the larger issues of postnatal depression. But that interest was aroused, absolutely, from the physical and emotional experience that I suffered. Most of all, I felt betrayed: my depressed mood was completely dislocated from the socket of my happy circumstances. Baby blues be damned – this was like the end of the world! The tragedy of postnatal depression is perhaps not the granulated horror of what is experienced in your mind and body, but its foreign surprise – one does not spend nine months, after all, preparing for a boxing match with the devil, we spend that time in joyous anticipation, if all things are well. Further, it is the consequences of the depression, and our unpreparedness that have the direst consequences. How does one live with the knowledge that you have squandered a happiness never able to be had again?

My list of felt and lived horrors, with this first bout of depression, would include dealing with the certain pull that the edge of the cliff held for me as I walked around its edge, the ocean killing itself on the rocks below, as Ulrike was safe in my pouch. This is why I never walked alone without my baby girl – I needed a greater duty to stop my indulgence. I began to know what silence tasted like. I felt sure that neighbours were spies, reporting my failures to an authority. The man in the video shop, ditto: I stopped talking to him as I hired out too many movies every day. Friends visited, but I could not understand their chatter, nor why they did not take my baby away with them when they left. My daughter did not like me. I could tell by the way I made her unhappy and full of tears, and I was unable to name her for six weeks. And the worst thing? Nobody except me seemed to think I was going mad.

On the surface the 'system' was a good one, with enough checks and balances to ensure that caregivers were doing what they should and could. A community midwife visited three times at home, following our release from hospital. After that there were compulsory visits to health centres to have your baby weighed and check up on mums. I had friends and family who visited. However, I spent my entire time trying to impress one and all with my ability to cope because I was so monumentally ashamed that I wasn't coping. I remember once it being a task too far to have to dress poor Ulrike again after I had undressed her at the health clinic. I started crying.

The nurse was annoyed at me for me making others wait unfairly. I got the message and curtailed any further subconscious cries for help. How hard can it be to dress your baby?

There is of course an accompanying list of 'reasons' and factors that contributed to my depression, if you want to let them onstage. I had not wanted to come home to Australia. We did not have enough money. Matthias was working two jobs, teaching in school during the day and at the Goethe Institute in the evenings, so I was mostly alone with a newborn for 14 hours or more each day. I had my first book contract and the book that was not finished was overdue. And past traumas were taking on the role of shadow puppets in my daily life – I was still very angry with my father for his alcoholic intrusion in our life in London when I was freshly pregnant, for his empty liquor bottles and his rude accusations of me being a poor daughter. A few other things like this need to be added to the 'causality' list, because they felt like fresh wounds rather than ancient history. This is why I write poems, I suppose, because they explain things better than lists.

When Matthias had lost his job in Sydney due to a restructure, and our world caved in, there were nonetheless some very positive repercussions. I will never regret moving north to Lennox Head, or that Ulrike spent her earliest life with the ocean as her lullaby. As soon as my life had been restored to this 'prestigious' pattern of being a woman who worked, with an employed husband, and a baby in the hands of a fabulous nanny, I felt safe and was happy again – or so I thought. Happy enough to go swimming again without worrying that I might aim for New Zealand and not bother coming back in, that is, but not happy enough to stop chanting my secret prayer *I want my life back I want my life back*. Someone, somewhere, heard my prayers. On the plane to London I said Take that! to the universe, and it soon paid me back big time for my insolence.

MISCARRIAGE, AND THE END OF A MARRIAGE

Life in London this time around was dreamier than ever at first. I was sleepwalking with joy. What a place! What a job! And with the job came a fabulous little flat in Mecklenburgh Square in Bloomsbury, complete with a locked private garden to access, a health club with a pool and next to Coram's Fields, that fabled children's playground.

The university less than 10 minutes' walk away and Ulrike's new nanny lived five minutes away. What more could I want? In fact, walking Ulrike up and down the beach as she slept in her buggy, I used to chant and pray for exactly what I had been delivered. Dee, Ulrike's new nanny, is another woman on my list of pleas for saint-hood, so we were very fortunate to have found her, and everything she has done for us and our family since. Matthias landed a job as a teaching consultant which paid well but never made him happy. What made him happy was the news that we were to have another baby – I told him over lunch one sparkling summer day in an out-door restaurant just off Oxford Street. Even my boss was genuinely happy for us. So what was my problem? Perhaps the first inkling of my suppressed fear was voiced by my professor's then wife, who upon hearing my news let her true thoughts be known. Having popped in for a cup of tea, she came into my office and gave me a loud, hearty lecture about my lack of consideration for the academic team that made up the Australian Studies Centre. Who did I think I was getting myself pregnant when I was meant to be covering her husband's absence on sabbatical? How did I think I was going to maintain a suitable research profile with babies to care for? And travel all over Europe promoting Australian studies, as was my duty? Years earlier, in between my undergraduate and postgraduate studies, I had won an editing job at my university, and this same woman had not. Clearly, she was still resentful, and said as much. She proceeded to tell me that I was too big for my boots, and did not deserve any job, and that she had warned her husband what would happen. I was a saboteur. I was trouble with a capital 'T'. Before flouncing out she reminded me that smart girls get nowhere in life, and let me know that it was she, not her husband, who had graduated with first-class honours. She left. Despite the paper-thin walls, which meant that everyone heard this tirade, no one came to offer me comfort, or contradict her enraged commentary. I did not cry. I went on with my work.

From this distance, I am able to see the cracks that were there in this 'perfect' life, but not visible to me at the time, like the silent sexism of the profession, and dealing with the mad professor's wife. In 2005 I went back to London for a working visit, taking Ulrike with me so that she could visit Matthias in Germany after catching up with friends and family. Apparently, people had their own ideas about me, and how I had 'coped' with life, as my diary reveals:

JANUARY 2005

Dear Diary

I've just finished giving my last ever paper at the Australian Studies Centre. It has to be my last. I was talking about Nikki Gemmell and Susan Johnson, and how they write about London in their novels. How they write about being mothers, in the cosmopolis, a long way from home. About how the freedoms of artistic life in the capital remain an intense pull for women writers, and why that might be so, even in these postcolonial times. I suggested that it was about feminist desire to be unknown, and free, and to write without constraint, and that this was still not possible in Australia. A bit of a dud paper by all accounts really. I don't think, without the exception of one recent ring-in from Australia, anybody had read any of the texts I was discussing. Maybe I am boring. Certainly, I bore myself. I wanted to write a whole book about Australian women writers in London. Now, I think I'll just write a book. Ulrike is asleep. We had a late pizza. Dee was babysitting. Her old nanny! She shocked me, having a laugh, talking about when she worked for us as a nanny, 'What are you like! Never met a mother like you. Met me on the university steps. Throws the baby at me. See you later. Ta ra.' God. The pain I was in. The pressure I was under. I think, if I have to be away from my babies my whole life long to work, I might as well write, instead of writing about people who write. She's asleep. Tomorrow morning, Heathrow and home.

What am I like, indeed? But Dee was right. Matthias and I had been under enormous pressure, returning to London. I had to begin work immediately, and it was a job that demanded being free to attend official functions in the evenings, which turned out to be so regular that I had to stop breastfeeding. Matthias's job was being held open for him until we found childcare. We had been wrongly lead to believe that a nursery place was being held open for us. By the time we found Dee, we were broke again, and I literally thrust Uli into her arms and rushed up the stairs to the university, late for a meeting, as the bus had broken down in Islington. All these things and more: these are the sins that I lay on the floor crying about, years later, unable to get up. For two years, I slaved at my job, trying to earn my right to be there. I was a lucky girl. But I felt like an imposter – I went to Richmond River High School, on the wrong side of town, for pity's sake. Then, everything fell apart.

It is a small story, really, what finally undid me, and rendered obvious what a lie of a life I was really living. One day I was pretending to be me, the next, there I was: me. James and I were extraordinarily close friends when you come to think of it, for two people who rarely saw each other and made no contact with each other between meetings (we both served on the Executive Committee of the British Australian Studies Association). One night, after not having seen each other for almost half a year, we were standing together at the drinks table, upstairs in the magnificent Downer Room at the Australian High Commission. It was an atmospheric room, both warm and grand, full of the happy ghosts of Christmas parties and play readings and political import. Les Murray was reading from his fabulous verse novel, *Fredy Neptune*. We were hosting him, and for some reason there were fresh asparagus sandwiches on offer (I think our committee president, Ruth, farmed asparagus in Sussex). James asked me if I was coming out afterwards. 'I don't think so', I said.

I'm pregnant, if you haven't noticed you moron, I have to go home and sleep. I'm done in.

Jesus, so you are. Sorry. God. Congratulations.

Thanks.

You don't seem too well, now you mention it.

I'm OK. It's just all been a bit of a shock.

I know what you mean.

What?

My wife's pregnant too.

But that's great!

Why is it great for me and not for you?

Don't be a bastard. You know what this job is like. They're not exactly happy I'm pregnant.

Well. They will keep giving women jobs. Ha ha.

Yes. They will. Did you know, his wife took me into his office and told me I was ruining 'Her Husband's' life, that now he wouldn't be able to go on sabbatical and finish his book? I didn't know what to say. Particularly as 'Her Husband' had been so happy for me. Very odd.

I certainly would have known what to say to someone who spoke to me like that.

She wouldn't have said it to you.

I should hope not. Men don't tend to get pregnant.

Lucky you.

Hey. Susie. It will be all right. This is not the dark ages you know. We do have something called maternity leave, haven't you heard?

Fabulous. That makes everything all right then.

Go on. Go home. I'll sort things out here. I bet Matthias is overjoyed.

He is. Are you? Overjoyed.

Not really. No. You know my wife's been having an affair.

Charming. Wow. Sorry.

Yes. Wow indeed. I love babies. I'm just not sure this one's mine.

God. Sorry James. Listen to me moaning! Sorry.

Don't be. I'm sorry you're not happy.

I am. It's just that things were so hard last time. I feel like I am about to lose everything. I didn't write my PhD to stay at home and change nappies.

Nevertheless, you should go home. Go on. There's plenty of people here to look after Les. And you've got to run the Les Murray extravaganza all weekend. Go home. Damn you. I have to find someone else to have fun with now.

I went home. The next morning, I went and opened up at Russell Square nice and early. The symposium had a wonderful atmosphere. Sometimes Les would listen to people giving papers about him and sometimes he'd slip off. At one point he came upstairs to my office and wrote his first ever poem on a computer. We cursed the automatic capitalisation at the beginning of sentences, as I didn't know how to turn it off. But I couldn't pay proper attention to anything. All day long I was spotting. It began as small spots, as though I had pricked my finger. By midnight, after hours of seeing small golf-ball-sized shapes of blood and gristle fall out of me, and bleeding so much that even using Ulrike's nappies didn't work, I passed out. The ambulance ride was silent and I was floating. At 3am I nearly died. One minute I was lying on a table with lots of medics around, joking, debriefing about their Saturday night's work and all the patients they had seen, and the next someone said, *she's going down*. After that, I was above them all. I was so worried about Matthias. I couldn't help him. I couldn't get back down.

I didn't die. The next day, when I woke up after surgery, they told me I had lost the baby. I already knew. It wasn't the hours of labour delivering clumps of horror. I saw my baby leave. And I had tried to chase her.

Then came the crying and the bereavement that cost me my marriage. Then came James. Had we made that baby die, us and our talk? Despite knowing the statistics relating to miscarriage, or having become familiar with them since, this has done nothing to dispel my belief that the scene I related above cursed my pregnancy.

I believe that it was responsible not only for the loss of my child, but was also a large contributing factor to the demise of my marriage to Matthias. After James and I were married and had returned to Australia, in the process of making new friends and reacquainting with old ones, I sometimes shared this story. About the guilt surrounding my belief that I had wished my baby away. I always felt so very vulnerable, but the sharing was worth it. It seems I was not alone in this belief: more than one precious girlfriend has told me of very similar circumstances, and the subsequent feelings of guilt-tinged grief. Babies so often come to us when we believe the timing to be wrong. As I and my group of women friends age, we know enough now to pensively understand that perhaps it was our 'belief' that was wrong, not the timing of a baby competing for our attentions. Now that it is too late for most of my girlfriends to procreate, we have a different relationship to our history of fertility. For some this gives permission for a fresh sharing of stories and a chance to air our long-suppressed grief. Because miscarriage is not really spoken about.

Some statistics argue that almost 15% of first trimester pregnancies end in miscarriage, so that equates to an awful lot of silence for an awful lot of women, and men. Why such silence? In my case, feeling myself responsible, I felt I had surrendered my right to be regretful, and to express my pain. Also, miscarriage being so common, it is easy to underestimate the associated emotional problems, although postnatal depression statistics are reported in as high as 20–55% of women following miscarriage, depending on which studies you read for what country. Why?

I was inconsolable. I would feel normal, even back hard at work and presenting conference papers the following week (although I was very battered from the surgery and blood loss, and although I did not know it at the time, complications from this hospitalisation resulted in my early hysterectomy years later, so I was not physically well). Then night would fall, and my 'GG monster' ('Guilty Grief Monster') would lie next to me in bed and howl all night long. One night, Matthias had had enough. It was my baby too, he said. Fair enough. Why wasn't he holding me then? To this day, I believe if we had sought help, or if indeed either had been offered some, we would still be together. Perhaps that is my greatest folly, to believe this, but it is the only account I can offer of why we squandered our love, and divorced. Instead, he left me alone to cry. I buried myself in work, and life's mundane demands. Buying a house. Writing a book. Booking and taking holidays. My life was on automatic pilot, powered by blood that was not my own: I came to believe that the blood transfusion that had saved my life had also robbed my sanity. Certainly, it took away the Susan that I once knew best.

I was the perfect basket case, in many respects. I had not properly accepted the loss. I was suppressing the grieving process – even though I could not control my night sobs for about five weeks, I was fully functioning otherwise, and in denial. Most people I lived and worked with had no idea what had happened. I deliberately did nothing to lose my pregnancy weight. Instead, eventually, I reinvested my emotional energy in a new relationship, a relationship with the partner of my guilty secret, James. He had been the only person I'd been honest with. When his baby daughter was born, we started speaking again, very tenderly. He had not felt able to contact me when he'd heard of my miscarriage, but later confessed that he felt our conversation had created a curse.

Some might say that it is not very sensible or helpful to peddle such stories, and that sharing secret beliefs like this plays no part in recovery from postnatal depression. For me, long 'recovered', only last week when I was expressing reservations about redrafting this chapter with a girlfriend over coffee, it was confirmed once again that it is an important thing to do. I had gone to school with this lovely friend and our high school had just had its 30-year reunion (much to our mutual shock) so we had a fair amount of history with each other. Nevertheless, when she pushed, asking me if it was hard revisiting this material, I was honest. Yes. But also no: not if the cost of the confession for me will be worth something. Why else would I be revealing such intimate details that will affect the characters in my story? I told her, for the first time, of the guilt of my miscarriage and the facts as above. Then she shared her story. And some other stories that I had never known. I went home a little more healed. I went home to finish this story for you and to wish that I too had a grave for that baby.

My children ask me about the birthday of their lost sibling. I'm not ready to tell them the full story yet.

Chapter 3

New babies, and the sickening punishment of genetics

I was seduced away from the life I had been living not by drugs or doctors or work, nor indeed my own depression. I was seduced by the idea of the future, and what might be possible. One day Matthias said he was going, and suddenly, almost instantaneously, I closed a door on what had once been. Without exchanging a single physical intimacy (despite what our divorce papers claim) James began what was nevertheless to become for me the seduction of the century. He wrote me love letters. He won my heart with words, confessing our lives to each other on a daily basis. I surrendered my 'sullied' self to him; in return he kept my secrets and married me. It was as though I was living on pure quicksilver. My whole life changed, and I wanted nothing more than for my grief to be gone and to be touched by the future. We planned to invent a new kind of colour. To write a history of love. To holiday on the moon. To create a 'supermodern' kind of family that embraced all comers. We planned for his ex-wife to be his best man at our wedding, for the children to know no pain, and for the oceans to become clean. We imagined everything would all work out for the very best. Who really knew what the 21st century would bring? We married as soon as possible after our mutual divorces and became pregnant with Scarlet almost immediately. Soon afterwards, our lives changed with an enormity that we had imagined but not calculated, forever. Let's just say things did not work out quite as we thought.

So many times I have tried to write what happened the day that Scarlet fell into a coma. If you navigated all that I have published since, hunting down my 'writing mojo', this life event is both a topic and an indirect theme in almost all of my writing since. So far, this story has let you into the 'secret' contributing factors to my postnatal depression, but Scarlet's (and, later, Hunter's) genetic illness is perhaps the most singular defining feature and distinctive characteristic of my nervous breakdown. It helps me to fictionalise what happened. Here, below, is a dramatised account of a child's collapse. In this little drama, the child, Marigold, dies. The Mum, Kat, and the Dad, Taylor, have been slightly neglectful in that they did not handle things as best they should. Go figure.

FROM 'BLUE LIGHT SERENADE'

They'd had a little party back at theirs after the christening, which had turned into something much groovier than Kat had wanted. The music and the grooving and kissing went on till way past Kat had gone to bed with Marigold, who were both truly worn out from the day and did not even enjoy their bath. Fractious girls together, mother and daughter surrendered, sleeping in knickers and nappies and not much else. Sleep blessed them, like a wisp of an old Seekers song promising the sandman with lanterns full of sleepy dust. Kat woke first to the sound of Taylor vomiting, and it was then that she clocked the silence from the cot beside her bed, and the fact that it was 3am and Marigold had not woken for her midnight feed. Taylor had seen the bedroom light go on and called out to Kat for help, sounding desperate. Kat picked up Marigold whispering mummy love to her, and Marigold, already wet and smelly from vomit, spewed again over Kat's silky gown, and started shaking. Kat nearly slipped on the gutter of vomit surrounding the cot, cursing, praying, crying, and ran with Marigold in her arms to Taylor in the bathroom. She was not feeling so well herself. Taylor, sitting on the shabby tiles of the bathroom floor – it was next on the renovation list – diagnosed a vomiting virus. Food poisoning? No. Marigold only did breast milk. They stripped each other off. Taylor held Marigold and told her the story of how she was conceived while they all tried to stand under the stingy shower together. Marigold was sleeping again, and Kat stripped and changed the cot, wiped the floor with disinfectant, gathered their stinking clothes, and put the whole grotty mess into the washing machine on 60 degrees. Kat got into bed with Marigold and smelled her beautiful baby head, singing a German lullaby that an old boyfriend used to sing to her, to the unfortunate accompaniment of Taylor having another vomit. He was sure it was only a 12-hour bug thing that was going around, so they'd all be OK by this time tomorrow. 4am. Marigold had refused milk, but drunk a small bottle of water. 5am she had vomited it up again. 6am Taylor took some drugs, and fell into a deep sleep. 7am Marigold vomited all over Katarina again, Kat was wondering where on earth all this was coming from, and put Marigold back down even though she was looking very sad, and blank, while she cleaned up, and ran a bath for them. Before she hopped in for a soak she checked on Taylor, who looked ashen and was dead asleep, and Marigold, who looked as white as Queen Elizabeth, her little body was limp and still but there was a determined glaze in her eye. Kat hesitated: should she pick her up? No, she decided. I stink. She's not crying. She needs to rest. So she tiptoed out, and put herself in the bath, and spent far too long in there, relaxing after she'd expressed the excess milk that Marigold would not take, wishing that Taylor would wake up and pick up Marigold now that she had started to whimper, as she was tired to her marrow. 'Taylor?' No response. Exhausted, bordering on the irrational, Kat was feeling only anger as she went in to check on her demanding baby daughter. Kat picked her up, and sat in the rocking chair with her. As she unfastened Taylor's big daddy bathrobe, and tried to get Marigold interested in her breast, she noticed that the corner of Marigold's mouth was curling. It was ugly. Terror came. She put her back in the cot. 'Taylor Taylor Taylor wake up'. Taylor woke up but only to go and vomit. Bloody men bloody bloody pissweak men, thought Kat. Get a grip. Kat pulled on a pair of old jeans and a jumper without a bra, then thought better of it, you never knew what was going to happen in the hospital. She dressed again. This time with knickers, a bra, a T-shirt. She packed the baby bag. She put a book in. She found her car keys. She threw some clothes at Taylor as he tried to crawl back into bed. Get moving she said, Marigold needs to go to hospital. They fought. He was loudest, but she was maddest. Her lip is curling, Kat said, why does she look like that? Taylor grabbed Marigold, and was out the door before Kat could find her wallet. She wondered if she had time to look for some lipstick. She walked outside, no shoes, she was freezing. He drove, she held Marigold in the front seat. They did not wear seatbelts. Taylor was at the hospital in the doctors' car park within five minutes. He had to stop to vomit. Kat ran ahead to emergency with Marigold. She had forgotten to do her jeans up, and kept tripping. She ran through the doors and almost dislocated her shoulder. She screamed out that her baby was dying, thinking as she did so how melodramatic, what a fuss, I am sure to be embarrassed by myself any second. Marigold now had blue lips, like bruised pansies. She got to see the triage nurse immediately. Before Taylor had even found where they were, there were three people standing around the now unconscious Marigold. A woman asked her how this had come to pass, and Kat could only weep at the sight of Marigold stretched out on the hard bed, strapped down, already ventilated, doctors extracting blood. You are taking this really well, she said, the doctor. The doctor had her hand on Kat's shoulder. Like a plant trying to pretend it was not your parasite. That's when Kat started to shake. What? What am I taking really well? Taylor arrived. He was all through vomiting. He told the story. A decision was made that the thing that was seriously wrong was probably metabolic, so when they phoned through for the transfer to a paediatric intensive care unit they asked for Great Ormond Street, who were best at that, apparently. Kat watched them trying to put a tube in and failing, and then cutting a hole in Marigold's inner thigh as though murdering her to finally insert the thing. Such trespass. *You are taking this really well.* Her back was turned away now, she did not want Marigold to open her eyes and see the horror in her own. *Really well.* The emergency team arrived from GOSH. Katarina felt the most deeply political she had ever felt in her whole life at that moment, thinking, suspended from grief like a hooked fish on a high wire, that the NHS does some things extremely well. She was proud to be English, grateful to be a Londoner. Absolutely amazed that she could be thinking such rubbish at such a time. Taylor was not thinking anything like that. Taylor was thinking, Marigold will be fine. Taylor was also thinking, Kat will not be fine. Taylor was thinking, Kat is reed thin on the sanity front. During all this, they did not hold hands. They did not look at each other. They did not talk. They did not ask questions. They stood, behind the crowd now working slowly with deep accuracy on the tiny body of a child. Their child. Marigold Marigold where are you? There was some kind of maniac in the next room screaming revenge at the casualty staff for not issuing him the drugs he wanted. Taylor wanted to shoot him. They were so very slow. The doctors were now moving with a solid, slow precision, with a glacial determination. They were gone for three years taking the X-ray. Then another five before the lead doctor from the rescue team said OK they were ready to transfer. Kat was held back when she tried to follow, as though by bouncers, she a drunken wannabe in the queue at China White, late in the Soho night. You'll have to make your own way down, they said. There was suddenly a social worker. Taylor told her to fuck off. She left. Everyone was silent. Marigold was gone in a squeak of trolley wheels. Everyone else left, their hugs were brittle candy, torture.

Taylor took Kat's wrists, and looked into her eyes. He walked her out, not letting go. Forgetting their car, for some unknown reason they walked home. Without speaking, they went into the house, and packed an overnight bag. Taylor lay Kat down on their marriage bed. They cried. They left as soon as they heard the horn. The taxi was waiting outside, and when Kat said 'Great Ormond Street Hospital for Sick Children' please, and Taylor said that it would take longer than she understood before they'd be allowed to see Marigold in intensive care, the driver did not say another word, drove softly and expertly through every red light, and did not charge them, said to donate the fare to the hospital. This is an excellent day for London, thought Kat. This is not looking good, thought Taylor, a little later, as he saw the medics stop talking as they buzzed their way through to the high security section into the intensive care unit. Not good at all. Taylor turned to Kat and said I love you Katarina Saltbush I love you to Bronte Beach and back, deeper than the Pacific, I love you bigger than the oldest tree in heaven. Katarina kept looking into Taylor's eyes. She would not could not move to where the staff tried to get them to go. She fell to her knees. She knew. Marigold had not made it across London. By the time the results were back seven weeks later, explaining Marigold's death, Katarina was also dead.

The above is, as I said, fiction. I can pick the real eyes of it out for you, of what I felt, of what it feels like to believe your child to be dying. When Scarlet was in intensive care at GOSH, you soon came to understand that while it was an extraordinary experience, there were plenty of people in that small geographical space who spoke your emotional language. Talking to other parents in PICU about what it is like to have a very sick child is like no other conversation. Or to a parent of a dying or recently dead child – and, it is a curiosity, but people in the latter category, these parents of dead children, they give you honorary membership of this A-list grievers club, or at least a day pass into the long room, as though your flirtation with their experience, your 'almost-thereness-but-for-the-grace-of-godness' is worthy of their pain. They will talk with you like with no other about what it is like to be so utterly helpless, watching your child slip away. We share a common language that is only spoken by those who have run over a snakoe and killed it, and are at one and the same time the snake beneath tohe tires, dying, or the snake curling its way around the crankshaft waiting for its own fear to allow it to kill you. They are mystical, nonsensical, vital, shared narratives. It is a courtesy too far, this inclusion. It is such conversations that saved my life; it is this language that remains my truest tongue. I have two close friends who lost a child. One of these, a woman who was around at the time and went through each day of Scarlet's coma blow-by-blow, was the only friend who really understood me, and all my subsequent behaviours, and forgave all. She also scooped Ulrike up into her own large family, and cared for her devotedly. Other family arrived in London and offered sterling help of all kinds, but it was that girlfriend who understood without question why we might need to have a long chat about the various virtues of cafes near GOSH, and other more scary topics, years after othe event.

It is not hard to locate the metaphor in my unfinished novel. Katarina dies (she suicides) because, metaphorically, that is how I felt. Whatever happened to me when Scarlet was in a coma, I am not certain I recovered. Something, akin to a death, altered me, irrevocably. If I felt embarrassed by the self-indulgent (so I believed) nature of my grief over a miscarriage, then I was about to embarrass myself on a completely new scale with the 'indulgence' that a nervous breakdown entails. But, that was still 11 months away.

The acceleration leading to that massive collision of health and sanity began, though, with what seemed an innocent enough health scare. I was 20 weeks pregnant with Hunter, and Scarlet had just turned 9 months old, when our whole family fell ill with a vomiting virus. Whilst trying to feed Scarlet, I noticed what turned out to be signs of febrile fitting (the curled lip), and had had enough experience of babies to know that this was not normal, not something to 'shrug off'. We dressed, woke Ulrike, and James dropped Scarlet and me at Emergency (Homerton Hospital was very close to where we lived in London's East End) whilst he ferried Ulrike to the girlfriend I mentioned above. Friends. By the time he returned half an hour later, Scarlet was in a coma and her life was hanging on to one or other of the many tubes inserted into her precious little body. I literally did not know how serious things were until he walked into the room, full of more than a dozen people working on Scarlet, and one of the doctors came over to us and said that we were taking it all very well. She touched my shoulder gently. It felt like a condolence offered too soon. I remember feeling offended, just before I collapsed. At 20 weeks pregnant, I look like many mothers at term, so this collapse caused its own set of dramas. Meanwhile, that team of brilliant people saved our daughter's life. It would not be the last we saw of them by a long shot, but can I please say thank you, thank you for every night you studied too hard to get to and through medical school. Thank you all.

It was some time – over a month, due to the complicated blood tests – before Scarlet was officially diagnosed with MCAD (medium-chain acyl-coenzyme A dehydrogenase) deficiency, but only a few days before the metabolic team at Great Ormond Street offered the tentative diagnosis. It is a genetically inherited condition that at the time was less than two decades old in the 'textbooks', so we had no way of knowing that both James and I had the deficient genes, and that any children we would create stood a one in four chance of having MCADD. The condition prevents the body from converting fats to energy, so any periods of fasting are potentially life-threatening. People with MCADD, if they fast, risk serious complications ranging from seizures to brain damage, coma, and sudden death. All this can be triggered by periods of fasting, which often accompany illnesses such as viruses (for Scarlet it was always tonsillitis). As diseases go, it is pretty rare – in 2002 when Scarlet was born we were told by the experts that the rate was 1 in 17 000, but since testing at birth has become more common in some countries, this rate is sure to change. One specialist said to me that she believed MCADD was likely to be responsible for 90% of cot deaths.

Overnight, our entire world had shifted. Our baby daughter was in a coma with a rare and life-threatening condition. If she survived, she might suffer brain damage. The baby I was carrying stood a one in four chance of the same fate. Before Scarlet stabilised, the staff would sometimes ask us to leave if the tests they were performing were particularly intrusive, and lacking any will or autonomy I complied. I regret this compliance, like many of the decisions I have made on the long 'automatic pilot' of my life in the years since. But then James and I went and walked around Russell Square like zombies. The same place that I had once sat, pregnant with Ulrike, looking across at the Georgian building that housed the Centre for Australian Studies, before I walked inside to tell my mentor that I couldn't accept the job because Matthias wanted to go home to Australia. The same place that I gazed upon from my office window for almost five years after I won the job again a year later. So many lunchtime sandwiches, so many coffees, so many seasons. And there I was, walking on a familiar path that now felt so tilted that I stumbled with each step. The only thing I knew for sure, was that nothing would be the same ever again.

Scarlet eventually came home and thus begun our formal relationship with squads of specialists, from metabolic consultants to neuropsychologists. I am in such awe of these human beings. One day I hope to write a history of Peter Pan in performance and donate all royalties to the hospital. Meanwhile, we prepared for Hunter's birth. He was born in the fine English summer of 2003. It had been a rocky five months. James was working in a different city. We had a run of bad nannies, with all the unsettlement that entails, but Dee stepped in miraculously, until the wonderful Erica arrived in our lives. I was in a new academic job at a different institution and they were not happy that I was about to 'trounce off' on maternity leave. (In fact I never received a card, let alone flowers or congratulations or any sign of courtesy from my colleagues, which devastated me and made me very anxious about returning to work.) It soon became obvious that Scarlet's repeated hospitalisations and coping with two sometimes very ill children was not something that any parent in their right mind would leave in the hands of hired help. One of us would have to leave our job. As soon as this was understood, everything became clear. We could not afford a London mortgage, and care for our three children and support two others financially on one income. We decided to go home to Australia. This decision became destiny, as on the very day I was offered the job in Australia our cherished nanny was deported at Heathrow, on her way home from visiting family. I had never asked to look at her visa; the fact that her references for working with disabled children were impeccable had won her the job.

That was that. Shortly after Christmas we put our Hackney home on the market. I signed my contract on Boxing Day, and we were living back in subtropical northern NSW before the end of January. When we landed in Sydney, the first thing Scarlet did when we walked outside the airport was take off all of her clothes. It felt like paradise. Before we left London, our consultant team had encouraged us to pursue a life as we imagined it, healthier and stress-free. They reminded us that our spot in family therapy had just come available, to help us deal with the post-traumatic stress of Scarlet's near death, the diagnosis of two children with MCADD and its impact on the family. We knew we needed it – things had also been so very hard on poor Ulrike through all this – but we put the thought aside. The Pacific would wash all our cares away.

ARCADIAN HELLS

Seaside suburbia, and working in a regional university, did not turn out to be the paradise we had hoped. After a very short time at work, on the same day that Scarlet went for her first ambulance ride in Australia, those dreadful and so very harmful accusations were made against me which ultimately resulted in my collapse at work. Because of the nature of the way the allegations were made, and the conduct surrounding the allegations by my accusers, I was on paid sick leave, as my psychological injury was deemed to be one for which the workplace had been responsible. Certainly, this was what all the appointed medicos decided. The attacks were malicious and ongoing, and I had become so ill I could barely leave the house, let alone Lennox Head to travel to work. My life had become a round of daily medical appointments, sometimes even having to travel as far away as Brisbane and Sydney to be examined by the university's insurer's psychiatrists.

Then something strange happened. I was diagnosed by my GP with bipolar disorder after six months of not only failing to respond to antidepressants, but getting worse, despite his best efforts and those of various other therapists. The diagnostic penny dropped, it seems, after I reported having had a particularly bad weekend that involved being lost in the bush for half the night, with the grasses trying to talk me into 'coming away' with them. We happened to be away with my brother's family in what was my second only excursion beyond the confines of my seaside village and surrounds since becoming ill. The first had been to drive up to Lismore to the university, a trip that had brought on a severe panic attack coupled with vomiting. This time I'd tested my newly developed agoraphobia with a longish, five-hour trip to Giraween, a beautiful national park (aren't they all? – I've never been a nature groupie though) just over the Queensland border. The landscape is surreal, populated with giant granite boulders sitting atop deep bush. I felt menaced by this landscape from the second we arrived – even the herds of grazing kangaroos looked suspicious. While the kids, the 'Famous Five' cousins, got on with having a great time, I chastised myself for being strange, and tried to normalise. The children eventually crashed, falling into that kind of good sleep that only hours of bushwalking and happy exhaustion can induce. The barbeque had been of the best kind, thanks to the superior country sausages bought at the butcher in Tenterfield, and our outing to the local vineyards earlier in the afternoon.

Queensland is a surprising place. Once in London we were celebrating the work of the late poet Peter Porter, one of Queensland's best exports. Poets of the world would be unanimous on that judgement, I suppose. Anyway, there we all were in the common room of Senate House, post symposium, drinking a selection of white wine from Queensland, kindly supplied by the Queensland Agent General. The man from the *Times Literary Supplement*, rumoured to be living with an Australian and in the know about these things, made some good jokes about the safety of proceeding with drinking such an unknown and possibly dangerous, irreparable, drink. No one had heard of Queensland vineyards in London then. He was being cheeky, but it was surprisingly fine wine, and all too soon gone.

Anyway, I had advanced knowledge about those secretive Giraween wineries, and I had drunk too much on the first night in that stately, wild place. My Uncle Kev had always protested how good first nights anywhere were – fishing trips, excursions to the city for cricket test matches, holidays – nothing could beat the excitement of first night pleasure. It was a tradition that he filled all of us young ones with this excitement on many a family holiday on his farm. And there we were, living it all over again in Giraween. Over dinner, when it ought to have been time for a calming cup of chamomile and not another tankard or two of wine, I made the mistake of mentioning that a friend had been sounding me out about a job as a literary agent in London, news that my family took exception to. I remember taking exception to their exception – what had Australia done for me except, well, this mess I was in? Things went downhill from there. Next thing you know, hours and hours later, James found me and had to rescue me from those grasses and their murderous intentions. People die out in the bush. I was lucky I was found.

Telling this is both alarming and embarrassing – I was never so mad that I was not at the same time also ashamed of my behaviour. *Stand up, pull yourself together, and walk back inside the cabin. Go to bed you lush.* Anyway, the undergrowth's invitation was hardly impressive – where did those grass girls think they were going to entice me, down to Queensland's equivalent of the Groucho Club? Hardly. More likely into a damp creek full of wombat poo, for a bit of a mad splash. A girl has her standards. Is this what being mad is like? Am I mad? Who is going to take care of my babies if I am mad? Can I stop being mad? That is all that was going round my head, plus the fact that I desperately wanted to leave the scene of the crime – maybe the landscape was making me crazy?

Recounting these events to my GP upon my return, I found myself prepared for his proposal that I might have something other than your common or garden variety of depression. I had not been a student of literature for this long for it to go unnoticed that, historically

58

speaking, cut-snake madness was often part of the writer's package. Literary conferences – it had not failed to escape my notice – are potentially hazardous places. Morning teas, book launch soirées, and conference dinners are all places of operatic hysteria. Over the years I've seen fist fights, bitch fests and dysfunctional behaviours that would outrank any other group of professional people. And I speak as a long-time devotee of the Qantas Christmas Cabaret.

Aside from mad grown-ups, my youth had not been bereft of friends who had lost part of themselves through drug abuse, or were ripped apart by some deep grief or other. One friend, with whom I was lucky enough to work at K-Mart, busied himself saving me from insanity whilst he grappled with his own. As I was forced endlessly to tidy the boys' underwear section, he attempted to remind me of life's better logic by sneaking music we both liked onto the store PA system. We were addicted to the Masters Apprentices at one stage – *be who you want to be do what you want to do yeah-yeahyeah* – and could manage to get away with a few tracks before the manager noticed. He worked in the electrical section. He had manic depression. That's what it was called in the 1970s. So did his sister, and his mum. I only went round to his place once. That was enough. Sometimes he was at school. Sometimes he wasn't. Sometimes he showed up for work on Thursday nights and sometimes he didn't. He was in a band. Everyone was. One night on the turps followed by some dark poetic exchanges with gravel and grass did not, upon reflection, seem so bad.

The morning after my rescue in Giraween, I spent most of the time in the cabin's huge spa bath, with the kids jumping in and out and cuddling me. A little later I went for a walk across the paddock, and while my sister-in-law and I watched the kids trying to spot koalas in the trees, I felt her hand on my shoulder, and she said the kindest thing to me: something along the lines of *it's not your fault you know, Susan. You haven't even been diagnosed properly yet. When you do, then you'll get better*. So, following one of the worst weekends of my life, my doctor's 'have you ever heard of manic depression or bipolar?' came almost as a welcome relief. And that's when I was referred to Ian, my third psychiatrist, and the one who finally 'got' me. I started seeing him shortly before my return to work, and saw him for two more years, only stopping because of our move to Melbourne. He did not agree, nor do I now, with the bipolar diagnosis, but I can certainly see why it was offered, when you look at typical symptoms. Frankly, I think if I had been asked the right kinds of questions, things would have been different.

Something, like, what do you think is wrong with you? Or, what are you really mad about? Narrative medicine is fabulous, but who really wants a doctor who asks the kinds of questions I craved instead of one who can recognise a heart murmur?

WHAT THE GOOD DOCTOR SAID

Ian's official diagnosis of me was the one I feel fits best. I am very grateful for his complete openness in providing, unasked, copies of his correspondence about me to my other health providers. Reading these documents so many years later is shocking. I'm sitting here on a Melbourne winter's afternoon looking out at the gumtrees in the front garden, wondering if I can afford the emotional cost of writing this all out – I have to collect the children in an hour or so, and it's hard to dissemble yourself. *Susan has presented with a wide range of symptoms in this time.* I have to remember that I am well, that I can drive the car, and smile when the kids run out into the playground hunting down their loved ones. *She has a significant background history.* How far away from post-traumatic makes you safe enough to trust yourself? *She suffered with postnatal depression with each of her three children. She lost a child at 5 months gestation.* You think you have coped with all these things, then you read about them, you read your sadness there, documented, on a psychiatric report, and realise it is not done with. *There is a history of a somewhat unstable childhood.* You don't even work for the university anymore, and have long ceased to think of yourself as being vulnerable to professional sabotage, but still, when you read of yourself as having possessed *a sense of outrage at her experiences, primarily aimed at the university*, I go immediately back to that land of grief. When I read that *She has surprisingly little negative feeling toward the perpetrator of these allegations* I am relieved that my politics seems to have remained intact during those mad times. Still, I will always call her THAT WOMAN, not even worthy of a cuss.

Ian was smart about an awful lot of things that did not fully appear to register with everyone else that I encountered in my medical world. He did not even necessarily support a biological diagnosis of depression. *She presented as a tired woman.* Well, of course, as he knew, Hunter had been in hospital the night prior to our first consultation. *She is seeking meaning for what she is being punished for.* Any sensible person would, wouldn't they? Or is this in itself a craziness? *She has a degree of resolve about her currently, and I do not see her as a high suicide risk.* At that first consultation, Ian did not prescribe for me, rather he encouraged me to keep utilising my lifestyle antidepressants – yoga, surfing, and meditation – and to continue to engage in my academic and particularly my creative work. He emphasised that last point strongly. Over the next few years, we tried various drugs for treatment, ranging from antipsychotics to mood-controlling drugs usually prescribed for epilepsy, but the most therapeutic part of this relationship for me was the discussions, about what a diagnosis actually is, and what it can mean. So. Mostly I am me without drugs, except in times of extreme need. When would that be? When do you ever know that you are not coping? Experience shows the knowledge always comes too little too late – because of the speed at which I feel compelled to live my life.

JULY 2005

Dear Diary

I've been home from the UK less than a week and already I'm going completely mad. Last night was extremely distressing. My hand is swollen and bruised from hitting James. I hit him a lot. I am still lost and violent this morning and I walked for more than two hours to try and let it escape from me. As if. What's my excuse? That I've arrived home to a house full of children, not all of whom I can muster a fine kind of regard for, and his ex-wife, and my ex-husband, all living here, eating food I've paid for, messing up my world, and not giving a sweet Fanny Adams for anything but themselves. God knows what they've been doing all day while I've been at work, but certainly not hanging the washing out, preparing supper, shopping, making any remote effort to put the house in order, or for that matter, arrange Ulrike's transition to a new school, make a card for Uncle Graeme's 40th, blah blah blah. Listen to me. I put four of the kids to bed in a storm of silence. I had a shower. I continued to keep my mouth shut. I was shaking, and exhausted. By then it was dark and 'they' were outside fagging and drinking and I did my little-miss-prim number – 'Oh dear me, I do wonder what we'll possiblly be able to eat for dinner, what with all this lack of food in the house?' – (where do I get that from? I hate myself!) and locked myself in the study. Did two hours of online teaching despite having been on the road and at work for 12 hours already. I charged

61

them with getting food organised. Fish and chips, excellent decision. God I'm ranting. The story goes, they did not make it in time before the chippy shut. They came home with stuff to make that was going to take FOR EVER and make A HUGE MESS, and I started yelling and could not stop. Only the cruel comments of a man I can't even remember loving shut me up. I went back to work with a huge glass of wine, and left them to it. I ignored what I was feeling. Then all of a sudden I ran outside to them. I confronted James: how could he let my ex- talk to me like that? And then it was on. I was completely uncontrollable. All of the children woke up. Crying. It was a nightmare. I was a nightmare. I had to spend an hour, in shame, this morning answering repeated questions about why 'me and daddy' were fighting. Later I went into the uni and hid all day. And came home to a house that somehow spelt respectful co-existence, tidy and organised and harmonious. This was the thing that made me feel worst of all. It normalised my unforgivable behaviour, rendering it somehow beneficial to the household. It was not. It is not.

IS THAT ME IN THE MIRROR? COMING TO TERMS WITH DIAGNOSIS

Some months after the episode recorded above, I was sitting out by the swimming pool, having one of those beautiful working lunches that you can only have when you're married to someone in the same line of work as you, and that line of work is academia, and you have the autonomy to suffer the marking of hundreds of essays in whatever setting you choose. The table was cluttered with teaching materials, preparing for the week's classes ahead of us, and (mostly finished) piles of essays for marking. James was editing a manuscript. I was marking a postgraduate thesis. We fell to discussing the art of biography, and whether or not I might write that book about Sarah Churchill that I had been flirting with for three or more years now (Winston's actress daughter – it had originally been my notion to examine Clementine and Winston's marriage through the lens of their mutual mental illnesses, and the personal tragedies that befell them, but then I got hooked on Sarah's story). I said, I hardly think so, I can barely finish the one I'm working on now, writing about my own mad self.

We talked about work a little bit more, including the likelihood of me ever finishing this book, as I was so frightened of the revelations involved. James said: 'What is it like then? What does it feel like when you feel like you're losing it? When you're depressed and mad?' I couldn't say. I was lost for words. We sat there, looking at the pool, silent. He changed the topic, and said, 'Seven days now', and we talked for some time about how he felt about giving up smoking, and how he was coping. He said it was getting easier. I said, that's good. He said, he knew it would be easier every day. And then I said, that's not what it feels like for me. When I'm there, depressed, in mad land. I do not believe it will ever stop. I am, simply, possessed. And unlike the torture people go through fighting to end addictions, believing that they will be a better person for their efforts, I can never believe that something that graceful and life-affirming is possible. When I am depressed, I have no knowledge whatsoever of what I once was, or what I might become, only feeling the truth of the illness and its grip, which kills all vision.

We all of us have our bad moods. Our down times. Me too. But how do I qualify the difference between sad and ill, gloomy and sick, manageable bad moments and uncontrollable behaviour? How can I explain to myself let alone anyone else the different state of being? In the past, after and sometimes even during 'episodes', I have consciously tried to intellectualise what was going on with myself. To little avail. Since diagnosis, I have tried very hard to maintain an ever-alert interior monologue that cautions me at every sign of disturbance. I check myself, my mental state, as though taking a pulse. What happened on the night mentioned in the diary entry above was this: I knew I was in a complete state within five minutes of arriving home, and, consequently, I formulated the ambition to manage both the chaos and my own temper with grace and dignity. Be proud of yourself, I counselled, be a good mother. Be a kind host. Be Christian. Be especially nice to your beautiful husband, who has been most put upon of late. So how did I end up, within two short hours, beating him insensibly?

I knew I was very tired, and that this was often a factor when I lost control. I was also hungry, but events got in the way of me and food. I also said to myself, tonight it would be sensible not to drink, but this advice I completely ignored as I entered into the second phase of my anger. Insults trigger both grief and defensiveness in me. This happened. As I noted that I felt grievously angry, I stopped myself on my way outside to continue the fight, sat myself down in my favourite pink armchair, put my feet up on the matching ottoman, and tried to breathe. My blood was not my own. It had a foreign temperature, and my heart was doing a good job at pushing its new thickness around. I admitted: something chemical is going on. Stay put. Keep shut up. Calm yourself down. But the breathing, so familiar from yoga and meditation, only meant that I could hear the unbearable pounding in my head. I was coiled, and there was nothing for me to do but spring. I remained sitting in the chair, and watched myself losing further and further control of myself, and hitting and hitting and screaming and screaming. I was in awe of what I was saying – what pain that woman must be in, I thought. Then it was over.

I slept and I did not sleep. I got up very early, drugged with a depression that was constituted of gravel and deep mud, and forced myself to brace the wet morning and the beach. As I walked my arms and legs moved with some kind of fatalistic chaos, as though they were recent transplants from an unwilling donor. I had no coordination, and someone had stolen my mind, it was absent. I walked too far for health, until I was cold and exhausted, and then I had to face the long walk home. My body was marshalling, and now at last my memory was coming back, and there were some welcome tears of recognition. To remember yourself, even if you hate yourself and what you've done, is an act of grace. Is this how mothers love their rapist sons? Fathers their murdering daughters? I did not know. I made it home. I went to work. I did good.

REFLECTIONS

I was never really sure about my diagnosis. When I agreed to write this memoir, my first impulse was to phone up my psychiatrist and try to get an appointment somewhere between now and next century (you try living in regional Australia and being mad), so that I could ask him straight: Was I really mad? Are you sure? Can you tell me what it is again? How mad am I, exactly? Thing is, I got better. It had nothing to do with medication. One morning I literally woke up, went to my doctor and said I was going back to work, and that was what was going to make me better, fighting instead of giving in to my depression, and he agreed, and signed the forms that allowed this to happen – it turned out to be the right decision. I could not face waking up one single more Monday morning with my diary full of medical appointments, week in and week out. Hour after hour talking about myself. I was completely fed up, sick of myself. How people voluntarily stay in therapy for year after year is something I am only able to understand from Woody Allen's point of view, who, to paraphrase him badly, said that one day he just called a draw with his therapist and that was that. I said I was better. I was. Better enough. In fact, *there was probably nothing wrong with me in the first place* – or so I often think.

Let's just get this absolutely straight. After I lost my second baby my first husband and I lost each other, and soon after our divorce I remarried. In the first year of this marriage I gave birth to a daughter (Scarlet) who fell into a coma aged 9 months and was subsequently diagnosed with MCADD, while I was 20 weeks pregnant with Hunter, who was also eventually diagnosed with the same condition. We moved home to Australia, me taking a significant demotion, in order to care better for our family. *The move was precipitated in part by her children's health in London. Susan certainly feels it was not well thought through and somewhat rushed.* I'll say. And Ian didn't even know about our nanny being deported at Christmas time, unable to get back through Heathrow after visiting her family in Bosnia. In the context of so many people insisting that I was depressed, these facts do matter. *As you know, the situation has gone from bad to worse in recent months. She clearly lacks confidence in her employers . . . At the time of ongoing domestic problems due to her children's health, she was accused of plagiarism by a PhD student. While these claims were refuted by all . . .* STOP. All these secrets, and their sharing. It's not that it is all too much to bear. It is the opposite. Not enough – not enough about what really matters. What happened to me is simply the long trail of sewerage being flushed out into the wrong part of the ocean at the wrong time. The real toilet of this story is why it all happened, why I fell down. My baby daughter nearly died. I felt it was my fault, because I was suffering from postnatal depression, and not coping with much. Including her illness. As I write, the afternoon is seepage. The gumtrees are squabbling amongst themselves in the freshly arrived wind. It is time to find my keys and play mum.

THE FESTIVAL OF ME: THE PERFORMING PATIENT – SOME REFLECTIONS

I got better, it's true. But this is also true: when I am depression's whore, I am nobody's wife, nobody's mother. That, that is what depression feels like. When I tell (the few people I do) that I'm writing a book about having a nervous breakdown, their reactions are long, and generous, and curious. Often, many of the questions are about themselves. *What is it like? Oh. I think that happened to me once* has not been an uncommon response. Some people will tell you anything to qualify for entry into club mad.

My psychiatrist, Ian, has diagnosed me on paper as nothing more than 'cyclothymic', and often discussed with me how diagnostic detective trails of patients' failed responses to medications for depression, followed by revealed incidents of mania, can often lead to 'bipolar' conclusions. My psych has had long, delightful, life-savingly intellectual conversations with me about medicine and diagnosis and its art and possibilities – and failures. All the time, though, we were wandering like nomads through a long list of drugs on a trial-and-error basis – almost like prescribing to diagnose. And in desperate times, when I feel suicidal or murderous, and I am between prescriptive trial-and-error zones and have to see my GP immediately, I am always prescribed what I need most – antipsychotics – which let me sleep, and take me out of a manic cycle.

Of course, to be prescribed a listed drug for schizophrenia one has to be registered on the crazy person's database – try listening to that 'nomination' by your beloved GP on the phone to god knows what big brother as you sit rocking in their surgery. Valium. Please. Just give me some bloody Valium, and let me sleep, and let me be calm and work with it, and let Valium save my children from my worse self. But no. One can overdose on Valium. And I am a naughty girl, too naughty to be given what would work best for me. Why don't you try a different anticonvulsant instead, one that perhaps won't cause your head to break out in pineapple-ring-sized lumps?

I do not like what I write about myself. It is – post expression – almost unbearable to read. So, why would I expect anybody else to like how or what I write about them? This exploration of the doctor–patient relationship from the patient perspective (mine), which invariably includes writing about other, real-life people who were involved in my care, is I hope alert and respectful to the fact that the people I am writing about are not just healthcare providers. They are people, who, like me, will almost certainly not like what they read about themselves (at least their children won't have to read about them talking to grass). 'Respectful', she says. How respectful is any fight? What I am interested in, however, is that this argument does not become a shouting match whereby I win. Victory for the 'victim' is nonsense, especially if there is just another patient in the waiting room who is only one step behind me on the experiential trail. And there will always be more patients. Hurting people's feelings will do nothing to enhance doctor–patient relationships. So, what will? Am I ready to offer some considered and viable possibilities for improving the relational worlds of doctors and patients? I hope so. With apologies to all the characters in this story of care – and deep care it was – this is a narrative whose desire to be told outranks all of our combined egos. The perspective is mine, the festival of illness is mine, the performance of 'patient' is also mine. The re-enactment, then, is at my direction.

My summary of being ill, called 'Susan writes a summary of being ill'

» Susan was not properly diagnosed for far too long.
» Cognitive behavioural therapy does not necessarily work for people who think too fast, or people who prefer not to read books with pictures.
» Pride (on behalf of the medical practitioner) can complicate patient diagnosis and treatment, particularly when diagnosis and treatment is not going well.
» Return-to-work provision for those who suffer a psychological injury at work is a comic opera in need of ruthless rehearsal with a view to radical rewriting.
» Regional Australia is not a good place to be mentally ill.
» Doctors are time-poor individuals, impoverished in many ways, but this is not the fault of the patient.
» As an educated person, I expected psychologists and other psychoanalysts to be better read than me in the area of their own expertise. To perhaps know their Freud, for example. Or the history of women and madness, and writers and mental health. This proved to be a fantasy on my part.
» Susan does not trust doctors who have a less than competent understanding of the relationship between creativity and madness. Susan thinks in these circumstances you may as well talk to your dog. Susan thinks that any doctor who thinks it is OK to medicate you into a fit state to be a successful supermarket shopper at the cost of ever writing a poem again is not really making the patient safe, let alone well.
» We have staff meetings about difficult students, with the intention of caring best for them. I wish GPs could do this. Confidentiality is overrated. Seek help, and develop practices that foster such collegiality. Who would pay the bill for that conversation, though?
» It really helps to know what your therapists believe about therapy, and what kind of philosophical and intellectual position they hold about mental illness – what team do they bat for?

We need doctors . . . I respect them and their work enormously. Some days I wish I could be born again just to avoid having to live my life as I know it, and have 'real' skills. How much more satisfying it must be to be a midwife, just like the one who was in training and delivered Scarlet under the senior expertise of a no-nonsense Scottish superior, whose authority decided Scarlet's date of birth (she was born right on midnight). One does not mess with such people.

She had long caramel-coloured hair, the trainee midwife, tied back, and a soft, genuine smile. She was holding my hand. James had gone for a cigarette. The girl asked me what my husband did, and when I told her he was a historian, she told me her story. She had a First in History from Cambridge. 'Wow. What a change. Why midwifery then?' I asked. My contractions at that stage liked the breath that talking demanded. 'Well. My mum is a midwife. And so was her mum. And mum really loves her job', she laughs, 'Plus I absolutely did not want to go into teaching, urrgh'.

What a smart, sensible girl. What a beautiful touch she had, her calmness was enchanting. I envied her talent to study and understand and apply herself to this life she had chosen. A life free of the need to write books and extol the virtues of literature. The midnight arrival of Scarlet Rebel heralded her first delivery. How wonderful it must be to come home and sit down after a hard shift and know that you worked doing a job where you are still allowed to touch people, and that you help bring life into the world. The sense and beauty of it all leaves me awestruck. Oh to be possessed of the talent and wisdom to scrub up and make a better kind of difference!

I would never dream of complaining to a doctor. I would never dream of changing a single thing that has happened to me.

Chapter 4

Love and other addictions

Love can be such a squalid, selfish thing, but it is the very stuff of postmodern life. Does anything else really matter? Money, progress, humanity – they all seem so old-fashioned, somehow. Even spirituality is dated, being ultimately too individualistic. What is the meaning of life – is this the grit of all depression, to be without meaning in life? What I do know is that for me, exploring the subject of love, and sexuality, is essential to that quest for meaning, which is indeed one of the things I am grappling with in reflecting on these madder times of my life. Why is it that when all else disappoints, love is often the only thing that makes any sense?

Sociologist William Simon argues that in a world of continuing and continual transformation, sexuality is the ultimate postmodern discourse, because it offers no unifying thread to aid comprehension of our existence. That is, we actually know nothing about ourselves, and surrendering to love confirms this for us – what a stunning surprise love always is. Love is as unravelling as life. We embrace this unravelling, this unknowing surprise, because every time we come closest to our instinctual selves, we know how lost and unknowing we really are. So, as Simon argues, exploring the sexual and its dimensions occasions the opportunity to intimately consider how people deal with fragmented contemporary life. This sounds convincing to me. It would wouldn't it, to a writer who writes about practically nothing but, so I'm not exactly objective. Nevertheless, I propose that the confessional genres, by their very charter, should be confronting the reader with the type of revelation whose documentation creates the possibility for profound reflection. The chance, perhaps, to make sense. Or believe in the lack of it, which can also be a relief. So sorry, Mum, in the pursuit of answers, wondering if love is culpable, this is a 'knickers-off' chapter.

They say we are living in the age of the memoir, and despite my mistrust of the *zeitgeist*, here I am, telling you my sad little story, as though it must matter – some days, I feel I would be better off writing a memoir of my favourite dog, or maybe letting the dog write it himself. But if I am to persevere, I want to do this properly. It is no good, for example, talking about depression without serious consideration of the theme of love. What does it mean to tell this story, for me, for all the vivisection that this involves and the witnesses that will pay for it, for having been there with me in that landscape, with their eyes open? Unfortunate souls! I'm sorry if the telling hurts. Plato once proposed that all poets should be kicked out of his ideal state, because they all told lies. Where would they live, then, these poetic fibbers? Maybe they would live here, in the 21st century, in this contemporary world of confession, or in memory land itself, where everyone has something to say and permission, it seems, to say it. It is some theme park, this postmodern world. I'm sure the poets would eventually revolt and assume silence.

But for now, I'm talking, and this part of the story is about love, and sex, and marriage, and divorce, and how my intellectual as well as emotional relationship to 'love' almost predestined me to end up in a disappointing place, before things could change. All of my therapists had a lot to ask, and say, about my relationships. It is not as though, as a feminist and writer, particular in my plays and poetry, that I had not paid serious attention to this subject – or so I thought. I was well read, perhaps, but nevertheless emotionally illiterate. One benefit of having a nervous breakdown was that all the walls were down, and my gaze was honest. What did I see, and think about, the litter of my life so far? Serious depression affects relationships. Getting your groove back is hard. There are a lot of setbacks to recovery. Sometimes you find yourself standing up once more only to find that someone you had been leaning on has taken their own serious tumble.

I am also concerned, amazed actually, to read other postnatal depression memoirs, which all seem to go like this: I had a baby; I went crazy; I did not know how sick I was until [insert personal epiphany/tragedy]; once I surrendered to therapy and/or drugs I slowly got better; I am a better person for what I have been through despite the documentary of horror you have just read – followed by an index of contacts/services for those suffering from postnatal depression. All good – but this was not my story. I wish my therapy had been more productive. I wished I had been asked all the questions I wasn't asked and should have been. Questions like: why do you think this is happening to you? Is there anything you are not telling me? Do you think it would be worthwhile discussing your significant history prior to motherhood to try and better understand the nature of your depression? Do you blame anyone or thing for your mental condition? What do you think might make you better? Are you writing about this experience? Is this helping? What do you say on the page that you don't say in this room? What kind of therapy do you think would be best for you? Do you believe madness is a writer's lot? Or even, as U2 once famously asked, is it getting better or do you feel the same? Can therapists really tell when you are withholding information/being deceptive? How responsible is poor therapy for failing you? What makes a patient difficult, and what if they can't help it? What is a crazy woman to do with her list of mad questions that just cannot be answered by some doctors? I guess that's why I'm prepared to take you into 'the bedroom' now: too much shyness in the therapeutic process about this topic, about love, did not do me any good. Love, hopefully (it was definitely thus for me) made those babies. Having the babies made me mad. Love and madness are bedfellows.

One morning on the 73 bus, heading into Bloomsbury, reading the *Guardian*, I looked across at James's *Independent*. He was reading a much more interesting story. It was about the history of tattooing, or something, but it had a little side story about truth, and a comment about how tattooing allows us to conceal ourselves at the same time as asserting our identity. In the times when the upper classes thought it was fun to get a tattoo but bad taste to show it off, one Lord Redesdale, an English aristocrat of the 1920s, was told by his wife that the book *Tess of the d'Urbervilles*, which he had just finished reading, was not a true story. He was outraged: 'What? Do you mean the damned sewer invented it?' Our appetite for trespassing in other people's private lives is an insatiable desire, and it seems that the truer the story the better the fix – in fact, the less authentic the story, the less relevance its telling seems to have. But can we really expect a better class of truth about human relations from the confessional genres rather than fiction? And if so, do the writers of confessionals deliver the goods that their genre promises?

When my students ask me why I feel I have permission to write about, say, my family, and risk upsetting them, I have a set answer. I say, *because life writing is involved with the larger project of making sense of our humanity*. It's one of those 'for the greater good' lines that you'd expect an academic to say – predictable, institutional cant. I'm not sure I believe what I say, all the time. Writers write for money, for revenge, for ego, for love, because they can't stop themselves, for all kinds of reasons beyond the intellectual. In fact, intellectual rationale cannot even begin to explain motivations for writing a book, that primitive is the process. It is a primitive story, a story that can't be told without the tale of a baby that died, and a divorce, and the love that came and mopped me up. I never imagined, in the beginning, that it belonged to this tale, but it is perhaps the cornerstone of the whole fable.

To begin, here is me, falling in love with James, trying to talk myself out of it, writing a long list of reasons in my diary. I think I was using the 'second person' narrative style to try and be as rational as I could about the account I was writing. This diary entry was written by a woman whose depression following miscarriage had imploded her first marriage – as I've said, when I am depression's whore, I am nobody's good wife.

OCTOBER 2000

Dear Diary

That night in bed, deciding whether to say yes or no, you remember all the crushes you ever had. High school. Such beautiful surfer boys, so sexually talented. Then along came Peter and kidnapped you, trapping you forever in outer space with his death. Then all the others. You admit that Australian men had always been good lovers. Years later you are surprised to realise that this European desire for post-coital discussion is not your learned or preferred style. Having read too much Patrick White you are happy to believe that the planting of roses is more important than words. And there was such a long youth in that silent place, where the world was full of shearers, and you would fuck the first one who would look at you, when you were nothing more than a body. That was poetry but it is over. Then, there was the foreign surprise of the love of a stranger, he taught you your first language, the love of silence, so you married him. That was a great novel, but it is ruined, now, before the finish, killed by a twist in the narrative. So what is this, this bloody, thorned garden you have walked into?

You met him at work, in London, but he doesn't live there. After the board meeting, at drinks, you ask him if his wife is a vegan too and he gives a long answer. You are impressed. Soon you find yourselves deep in France together, at a conference. You are drunk and can't speak French and he is not and keen to get back to the hotel to phone his wife, but still, your talk is of the kind that lobotomises fear, and you know that here, in the middle of this wasteland at the end of the twentieth century, you have found someone more full of fat talk than you, with more composted, wild, beautiful, mournful ideas than poppies in Flanders Fields. It was settled within three blocks, by the time you reached Rue de Rivals, that you should write a book together. Your hotel. The chaste kiss goodnight that slipped. It was too late for both of you, by then. You go to your room, alone, that is what you want, and sleep falls away from you like the red sea parting, by your determined grief, as you cry, as always, for your dead child.

How do planes fly? You are circling Heathrow. Going home to you know not what. Your husband has decided. He is leaving you. And your daughter. England, and everything that has happened there, is too much to bear. You suddenly hate Matthias with a fury that extinguishes all memory of Santa Claus.

Another meeting. He had touched your back when he said hello, you can still feel the heat of his hand, and you lean as hard back into the chair as possible to increase this pleasure. Another conference. He kisses you, unexpectedly, in the long line for coffee, in front of everyone. They all know you, these people from around the world, gathered here to discuss Australia. Your mild shock at this disorderly intimacy cannot properly register. You are too busy, you have a conference to run and an unsightly spot on your face to cover up. That night, you walk back across the Thames together to the university, to another obligation. You realise that you can hear again, and that your own deafness had been a secret from you. You take a phone call from your husband, he is in another country now, it is the first time you have ever spoken to him holding another man's hand. He wants to try again. It has started to rain. You remember something useless – that a surf is always worth it no matter what the weather. This crush of soft rain, you know it will somehow kill you.

These are the things you say to yourself: I must never reveal how I feel about James. I must stop being juvenile. I must let go of his hand. I must stop listening to his spells of stories. I must say something witty and change the topic. He has a wife and two children, a newborn baby. I must listen properly and stop staring at him across the foyer, across all these sparkling people in this sparkling place. I must circulate. I must remember that I have known him for ages and he wasn't sexy yesterday and I must believe this lie. I must resolve to never sleep with him but write a story about loneliness and pathetic desire instead. Most of all, I must forget forever that on the night before my baby died, I had confessed to him and him alone in the world that I wasn't very happy about being pregnant. I must ignore his promise, his wish, his prediction, that we are destined to make more. Babies.

He has seen it and you believe him, but you fill everyone's glasses and think about Africa instead. You hear his laugh across the crowded space, he is taller than everyone else, and his charisma has parts of other people glued to him in lopsided joy. You are in deep shit. You deny this, take control of your life, go to the toilet and change a tampon. Apply lipstick. Say goodnight. Go and collect your baby girl, you forget you have stopped breastfeeding her, where does all this milk and yearning come from?

From that day on, for a long time hence, all of your poems are for him. One day, you will get over it. But not then, that night in bed, when you had done counting all your men, when you finally decided.

My doctors and therapists always asked me about sex, no sex being a signature indicator for them of a depressed person. Fair enough. I never told them the truth though, that this human instinct to connect never deserted me, even during my worst times. They would have thought me truly mad if I had told them the half of it. I had been mad for love for such a long time. When did this dependence begin? Had I been squashing love and sex together in a confused mash all along?

More than a quarter of a century ago, I was 17 years old and it was the summer holidays. It still felt like the 1970s, but it was in fact 5:45am on a Friday morning in the January of 1981, and I had stayed up all night waiting for the local newspaper to be delivered. The *Northern Star*. My small city of Lismore (then 25 000 people strong) was half an hour inland from the coast, and yesterday afternoon, on that very road which lead most speedily to the beach, my boyfriend Peter and my best friend Martin were killed in a head-on car crash. The driver had been overtaking another car on a bend. And there on the front page was a picture of the accident. I wondered if it was taken when their bodies were still inside. It was impossible to tell, so concertinaed and sculptured was the car.

This was how I found out. I had a lovely little Thursday night and Saturday morning job in a 'this goes with that' clothing boutique in downtown Lismore. I had been there for some years now, and the income provided schoolgirl me with all the pocket money I needed for bikinis and clothes and petrol and fun and parties. Which, of late, involved a lot of alcohol. This particular Thursday night was going to be a big one. It was a farewell celebration for Peter and Martin, who were off to Cairns tomorrow to try their luck and make their fortunes on the fishing trawlers. Since leaving high school the year before they had both been working as plasterers, but only to fund their first love, music. They played in the same local rock band, The Elite. That night, they were to play their last gig in Byron Bay as a support act for a band on tour from Sydney. The truck that hit them as they sped too fast back into Lismore to change for the gig before heading back down to Byron was the very truck carrying the band bound for Byron that they were to support.

All this, though, I found out later. In the beginning, it was like this: I saw the police car pull up outside the dress boutique I worked in, in the main street of Lismore. I somehow knew that inside the car was my father, a local policeman, and that he was coming for me. I headed out the back through the storeroom, and hid for a while in the toilet. How had he found out? Who had told him that tomorrow I was running away from home to Queensland, and not going back to school to complete my studies? I had not told a soul . . . except Helen. Was it Helen? No, Helen would never tell. My manageress was knocking on the door. I didn't want to see him, I said, please make him go away. Susie, Susie, come on now, come out. Something in her voice was unexpected, like a silver leaf in a mailbox. I came out. She already had my bag, and she walked me gently through the shop and out onto the street, and eased me into the front passenger seat of the police car. Dad was waiting. They said adult things to each other about making plans for my return. I was trembling. I hated him. I loved Peter. Then he told me. It was a black comedy of error.

Honey, I'm sorry to tell you this, but your boyfriend is dead.
Peter's dead?
Martin's dead, darling. Your boyfriend.
Martin's not my boyfriend.

75

Of course Martin's your boyfriend. He picks you up all the time.

That's just because Peter only has a motorbike and if he came to pick me up you'd freak.

Oh.

What do you mean he's dead? He's meant to be picking me up at nine o'clock.

He won't be picking you up. He's dead. Where were you going, what are you talking about?

What? What have you done with Peter?

He's had a very bad car accident. On the Ballina Road.

What happened? Is he all right?

Darling he is not all right, he is dead. I have seen him with my own eyes. Thank God I'd seen him with you or we still wouldn't know who he is. It's taken ages to cut them out.

So he's in hospital? You've got him out?

Yes, we've got them out, but . . .

Where's Peter?

Peter?

Was Peter with him? What time did this happen?

You weren't seriously going out with that druggy were you? I warned you about him.

Where's Peter? I need to see Peter. I need to tell him about Martin.

Honey, we haven't been able to identify the second body yet. You know all these boys then?

Was Peter driving? Can I see him?

No sweetheart. You can't see him.

At first I didn't understand. Who was driving? Was Peter dead or not? Yes, they both were. Much later I found out about their last moments. Apparently, Peter and Martin were doing their Peter and Martin thing in the back of the car, smoking grass, playing air guitar and drums. They died together. The driver survived, after overtaking another car on double yellow lines (no more yellow lines on Australian roads – surely my mood should improve with the colour updates!). I had to beg my father a long time until he told me how they died, how long it took. Did they say anything? He finally confessed, they died before anyone got there. It was instant. I knew this to be a fiction. But I needed to believe it, and I did, for many years. This poem was written whilst I was signed off work, absolutely sick at the thought of ever having to drive past that same corner ever again – a necessity, as it was the only road to the university. I really like Lismore, but it doesn't like me, alas.

When I was dealing with falling in love with James, and grieving my first marriage at the same time, I wrote a lot. Peculiarly, I wrote about 'young love', it became a preoccupying theme. Memories were coming out from within, like long suppressed bruises. It created some kind of comparative space for me, to remember myself decades ago, and compare the electric charge of my feelings in the current day. Depression had wiped so much emotional intelligence away from me, it was as though I could only trust the distant past as a reliable radar to gauge my current sanity, or otherwise.

'Damage'

I

I know I'm in trouble.
This has happened to me before
is still happening.
I can recall the bed,
the hand, the question
barely heard through the trail
his finger tattooed
on my back.
I was away from home,
away from love.
We had spilt it, ours, my husband and I,
and there he was, that man,
mopping me up.

II

There is a corner on a country road
leading out from Lismore to the beach
that I am forced to travel often,
that is well-covered with blood
and other ambitions.
It was a Thursday night and
he was coming to get me,
forever, when suddenly I was seventeen
and he was dead and
who wants to hear that old story now
the one that, still, twenty years later
tells me how to love? He's OK now,
I know, but I am not.

III

It is as if the man who knows everything,
the one who showed me peace and
took me there to be his wife,
is to be rewarded not in kind but
with the currency of the gutter.
He, who deserves angels, husband of a wolverine.
When my daughter was born he held her
for five hours straight and I, I forgot to ask.
It is impossible to ever recover from such a sin.

IV

It has been a very long betrayal
and I am sorry to have married and mothered
so often since, but in truth I lost love long ago.
You may find it asphalt deep in Molesworth Street
but it floods, that place, that town, it floods.
Or perhaps love lost me. Whatever. I practiced,
I am a diligent twit, but eventually numb, I gave up.
Imagine my surprise, then, to be taken back
to that ugly place. By you. Love swamp.
I know not the value of exhumation.

Growing up in the country, death was not something that happened elsewhere, or was easily concealed from children. Death was both high drama, and mundane. It was the overconfident drive home from the pub along the red gravel road recently graded after the wet that began with a death in a ditch and ended some weeks later in a shotgun hunt from the back of the ute for the emu who had consecrated the uncle's grave by scratching around the hump of dirt through the flowers, like a belated reaper. It was the priest who wore cowboy boots who had a sideline in outback tow trucks, who drunk too much beer at the wake and told you that this funeral was the first where he'd actually had to tow the car with the dead body back into town and rouse the bush nurse to declare the driver dead, then later preside at the ceremony for the dead. Death was the kind where old mother so and so was discovered dead having fallen from bed on her way for another bottle of sherry, and couldn't move because of breaking her hip, to be discovered when bachelor son number one gets back from the cricket in Adelaide. It was the girl who drowns only metres away from you, sucked down into the river by who knows what, with a million grown ups (or most of the town of 500) yarning on the river bank in the swelter, wide and warm from talk and sunshine and beer. Death was the grotesque canvas of the farmer's brains shotgunned out onto the wooden walls of the shearer's hut, don't want to mess up the missus's place. This is the work of neighbours, such deep cleaning.

I can't really imagine the things my father saw, the things he had to deal with in his nearly 40 years of policing. Cannot begin to. But we were always on the edge of this drama. We had, in those days of antique communications technology, what seemed like a small NASA command desk in our house. It was the police radio. When the coppers were out and about, Mum had to man it. Once, when there was a bank robbery in the outback town of Forbes and they were heading our way, through Grenfell and Dad was involved in the chase, the communications all became too much for Mum and she had to climb up on a chair in the kitchen to reach the cooking sherry. It was my turn then, flick the lever down, talk, *yes they just drove down Forbes Street*, flick it up, listen, flick it down and relay information to another police car. Over and out.

Another time we were all waterskiing at a policeman's picnic, at Bogalong Dam. The prisoners in Bathurst's high-security prison had chosen that day to riot, and every policeman in a hundred-mile radius was called in. All the men sped off so fast in the police cars that the dust from the gravel road ruined our barbecuing sausages. Women and children were left behind to finish off the day. We didn't pack up straight away, and when we did go home, the women were all tight with alcohol and light with merriment, scooping up sleeping children from dewy blankets. I got to drive a boat that day. Outback NSW was a very exciting place for a child in the 1970s.

The opera of Peter's promise and its legacy of wanderlust – what were we running away to, away from? – has only recently ceased to thrall, to hold me, but I still believe this: I am alive and they are not and I should live a life that somehow honours our imagined dreams. If it is only music, and love, that I can continue on with, then that is currency enough. My dear friend Martin used to sit in the playground at school and say to me, day after day, *have I told you yet today that I love you?* I chant this daily prayer to my children. I hope I never stop.

There were other deaths in my youth that mattered. Elvis Presley's sent me into a spin, for example. Peter used to play 'Love me tender' on the guitar. Then he died. Then Uncle Andy died of leukaemia when he was 36 and Uncle David suicided – more Vietnam vets have suicided since the war than died during it in action. Then there was Luke – well, you're asking for it, I suppose, if you're the third person on the motorbike and you're sitting on the handlebars driving home from a party at 3am. We all ask for it though. Hunter's godfather, Charlie, seemed to be forever in the Gulf, doing impressive things for the *New York Times*. I feel much better about him choosing Michigan, choosing a new life, choosing life: I hope he does too. Matthias doesn't ride motorbikes anymore. I was certain he too would die. But who am I to talk? When you wake up decades later, and you have the irrefutable evidence of a psychiatric report in your hand, claiming that you have a 'significant history', you have to wonder why. Was it something I'd done? Of course it was. For a start, I do not recommend taking hallucinogens before a double English class. Magic mushrooms and high school and teachers and John Donne are not a good mix. For a start, metaphysical poetry will never be the same again. To this day I cannot eat honey for fear that magic mushrooms may have been marinating in it – if my taste buds have been that affected, what about the rest of my brain and body? Sure, I had a fantastic time when I was young, but I do believe that my health has been compromised. And, I am not the only one who has had to pay for that.

Coming home to Australia with an English husband and children and introducing them to the landscape of my earlier life – revisiting the scenes of all my crimes – was an archaeological experience. I felt like I was being dug up. We drive up into the hills one Sunday morning to the Channon markets. These markets were the original 'hippy' markets, where it all began, the commodification of the alternative lifestyle. Nimbin is just around the corner, with its famous Aquarius festival history, where they all came for the weekend and never left, irredeemably changing the bucolic valley from dairy farming to what it is today. Scag city, the kids call it. In between all the communes and the dreams, the old timers remain. Deeper down the valley is Terania Creek, now world heritage, but in the 1970s it was the site of the biggest environmental protest in Australian history. My father policed there. I had to iron his shirts for him before he left. Then the hippies pissed on him from up high in the rainforest canopy. I was there, secretly, hiding behind the logging trucks, with Renae, who lived on one of the communes and went to my high school. Her dad was Californian. She was used to all this. Some political baptism. High times.

I sit in that same valley, in a different century, drinking chai under a huge canvas shelter, the sun abominably hot. The markets are big business these days, but aside from the fact that they are now a bona fide tourist attraction and thus have their fair share of visitations from the aliens of Planet Winnebago, not much has changed. All the kids are running around naked except for flowers, dancing to the band playing in the middle of the field. I am here with people I love. Except tonight, it is not the 1970s, and I will not be going to the village hall after the sun has set to continue the party, drinking magic mushroom tea from a cauldron and dancing all night to the band before driving home to Lismore with too many people in the car and uh oh going in the wrong direction and not realising until you'd crossed the Queensland border and only making it back in time for school the next morning by a baby's last breath. Again. No. I wouldn't be doing that tonight.

I was doing my very best to try and get better, but the past kept jumping up and biting my bottom. If I was so changed, why did the landscape look so time-locked? Why wouldn't the memories fade with my skin? This place was making me sick. I did not want to recall the way I had once lived and loved. Surely I was different now than when I was barely 17?

SATURDAY, 6 DECEMBER 1980

Dear Diary

On Wednesday night we had our school social at the City Hall. Peter's band The Elite played, and Martin's. We had a rage, but it was raining and a financial flop. It was a rip roaring punk success. Bringing everyone home got me into a lot of trouble, but it didn't stop Karen and Martin and Peter sneaking back to my house at 1:45am. Karen went home, Martin crashed, and Peter and I went to bed. We had an amazing time. His body belongs to classical Greece. The Elite sing a song 'Too pissed to fuck' but it's just a song. They left at 5:30. He said goodbye at the top of the stairs and made me nearly die. But I've learnt to keep my mouth shut and dream my dreams. Louise and I took Fi out for a drink and pizza last night. She's going to live with her Mum in Perth and there were tearful goodbyes but it's better than her trying suicide again. Then we went and saw *Superman II* in the new cinema in Lismore and were totally impressed. Martin's been around again looking for me. I was asleep. I want to go to their gig tonight but the olds are stiff. I could get around them but I don't know if I could handle seeing Peter anyway. I wish I didn't drink so much.

SUNDAY, 7 DECEMBER

I'm not sure I want to leave school. What I want is to talk to Peter. I have images of him that make me burn. Like when we were leaving the City Hall on Wednesday night. An empty, dark hall, I was sitting on the stage stairs and he was playing the piano in the curtained wings. Better than the gig. Martin said that's his sad song.

SATURDAY, 13 DECEMBER

What to ourselves in passion we propose, the passion ending, doth the purpose lose. What do you do when the passion won't go? Get pissed and sit in the top pub at Byron sharing a joint with a total stranger. I've left school. I'm going to go through with it. Cold Chisel are playing tonight and I'm bloody babysitting.

THURSDAY, 1 JANUARY 1981

New Year's Eve at Horseshoe Creek just past Kyogle with The Elite playing their last performance. Ended at 4am. Peter gave me a drum stick. Him and Martin rode all the way back to Lismore in Karen's boot. We all crashed at Peter's. 19 fucking 81. Shit. Time's a real arsehole. I feel slightly hung-over. He made me tremble all night. Julie came up from Coffs for a few days last week. We camped at Lennox and got extremely burnt and raged at Fowler's Lane, the open air Rock Spectacular! Yeah! So this year is going to be it. Here's to tomorrow.

THURSDAY, 8 DECEMBER 1981

Tonight Peter and Martin died in a car crash. *Reality is for people who can't handle drugs.* They were coming to get me. Dad came and told me at work. So sitting in the double-parked police car he told me that young Martin is dead. And his friend. Karen came up from Lennox at 1am. The paper came at 5am. There is a picture of the car on the front page. Drugs are a good thing.

I'm not sure if this kind of conduct locates the beginnings of what my psychiatrist meant by 'significant history of abuse', but why not throw this into the cauldron as well? There are so many things we don't want our children to do. Why is that? What on earth did my parents think I was doing? My room was underneath the house and had its own entrance. I guess they were busy with their own messed up lives: they divorced the next year. I had been binge drinking and worse for years. Hanging out with the local rock stars and staying out all night when you're still living at home, and meant to be in high school, and your father is the local copper, is not very sensible. It was very hard work, looking back, reading this diary. Believe me, I have saved you from the worst. Things got very ugly. And being 'home' with a foreign husband who knew very little about my teenage life, now a mother of three little children doing a bad job of it, I am not so sure it is a good idea to return to a place where you had once lived life so boldly that it overshadows any contemporary attempts to locate yourself within the same frame. Going back had been bad for me, in so many ways.

To this day, I have never stopped wondering if Scarlet nearly died because of me being a 'bad' person. All the women in my plays seem to be morally stained, or believe themselves to be. This is how I write my badness down. So I can focus on what matters. Gradually, the need I felt to take responsibility for my own life grew enormously, I felt it was intrinsic to my recovery. Owning the past was part of the agreement, ugly as much of it is. I have a whole trunk full of diaries that would serve any anthropologist well if they were interested in sex and drugs and rock and roll, Australian style, during that era. Is it over? Letting pathology take the rap for your own bad behaviour is boorish, the 'It wasn't me, it was my meds' kind of deception that is the refuge of the cowardly. Things that happened to you whilst you were young can mess you up. This I firmly believe. Things that you did whilst a young mentor-less adult may result in said trauma. This, I'm a living example of. More: as an adult with young ones to cherish and nurture, an ongoing abusive relationship with drugs or alcohol *etcetera* is frankly not a good look. I claim so often in my poetry that we are, all of us, damaged, and we are; but life is more quotidian than that; than poetry. Unfortunately. Someone has to cook the dinner. I like wearing aprons. It was time to put the past to bed. The first thing I decided to do was to stop wishing myself back in London, and appreciate afresh all the reasons why we had come home.

CHOOSING HOME, CHOOSING LOVE, CHOOSING LIFE

When James and I decided we were moving to Australia, after I had already accepted the job, we found out that it was not necessarily going to be easy for him to get a visa, despite the fact that we were married and had begat two children. He had to write a personal statement of his relationship with me, and have it witnessed by a series of people, including members of my family. It was a daunting process, writing our story down. Distilled, it went like this:

To whom it may concern.

I first met Susan in the autumn of 1998. She had just arrived from Australia as the newly appointed lecturer in Australian Studies at the University of London ... we hit it off pretty much straight away ... Over the next few years, I saw Susan frequently on my trips down to London, serving together on the Committee of the British Australian Studies Association. Often I would stay with Susan and her then husband. We discovered that beyond work, we shared other interests, including a love of loud, guitar-based rock music ... We also shared some intimacies about our lives which probably should have been an indicator of our mutual attraction. However, at this stage, and until October 2000, our relationship was platonic ... On New Year's Eve, 2000, I discovered that my wife had been having a long-standing affair with her boss. Following the birth of our second child in January 2000, she showed no inclination to leave her job. This seriously undermined any attempt at reconciliation. By September 2000, I realised I had fallen in love with Susan, who was at this stage separated from her husband. I told my wife I was leaving, and moved to London to be with Susan in January 2001 ... 31 July 2001, moved to Edinburgh to be near my children. 13 October 2001, married Susan at St Vincent's Episcopalian Church, Edinburgh. 5 April 2002, Scarlet born at Homerton Hospital London. 5 July 2003, Hunter born Homerton Hospital London ... Susan and I live our lives together fully. We have to be strong together to look after our children. Scarlet nearly died in February 2003 – she suffers from a rare metabolic disorder, MCADD, which was only diagnosed after she fell into a coma. Her brother Hunter suffers from the same condition. In dealing with this we've had to be strong for each other and strong for the children. And that's our life, a life we want to live in Australia.

Well we all know how strong I ended up being. James got his visa. We moved to Australia. I had a nervous breakdown. I got over it. Here we are.

JANUARY 2007

Dear Diary

I told my Mum that someone has asked me to write a book about being depressed. And asked her if she thought it was a silly idea. She said something strong and surprising and beautiful, telling me that I needed to write the book for all of us in the family who suffered. That it was important. That there had been too much drinking and alcoholism and pill-swallowing and violence and pain and suicide to be embarrassed about such things in our family any longer. That she couldn't watch the news without it making her cry, all the time, and that antidepressants solved this grief. That it could be everyone's chance to have a proper cry. OK, but I'm not sure if she'll still feel so positive when I've finished. Because it is not really such a dignified story, mine. And I don't really have a very innocent kind of depression, do I? Cowardliness extraordinaire is sneaking up on me.

Mothers, suffering from postnatal depression, are often guilty of concealment. I was good at this – too good, as women can be. Faking it for what, though? Looking back now, I wonder that love survived this time in my life. How did it? While I sometimes feel a little sorry for myself, imagining that when I was so violently ill I could have been better looked after – this is both a true and untrue wish – I certainly encouraged James, for example, to go and play cricket, for his own physical and mental health. But it was nevertheless costly for mine. I loved him, I wanted him to take some decent joy in life, and he loves cricket. But – I was on stress leave, unable to cope with small or large things. I could barely talk. I shook. And yet each Saturday during this period I found myself alone (abandoned to cricket by my husband, and cricket is a very long game) with three outrageously energetic children to manage. And I use that word judiciously, as they certainly weren't being anything better than that – managed. Not loved. Just herded, fed, and watered.

'Cricket'

Never mind, my love,
Soak up your sorrows
With cricket, I said,
And he did. And I ran
Along seven mile beach
So that I might find
My shadow before I fell off the earth
With my trip, it was tipped so,
That earth of ours, in those days.

Then one day I told him
How I felt about this strange
Saturday widowhood spent with
Feral children and my best girlfriend
Depression (she's always there
For me) and he went silent
And I thought, nostalgia warm, of that
Tricky kind of mud you find at the edge
Of a dam or by the irrigation channel
And I knew I was in serious trouble, the worst
Kind, the unoriginal kind, where you
Find you're quite content to steal someone else's
Epitaph for the sad demise of their own marriage:
I just stopped caring.

Part of depression is its culture shock. I have time for the series of
'travel' books, *Culture Shock!*, where either immigrants to a country, or nationals who have returned to their country after a long
period of exile, write a guide book about their country, its customs,
etiquettes and more. I wish someone would ask me to write *Culture
Shock! Australia*. I would have this to say about how architecture
turns the home in on itself away from the street, how huge double
garages vacuum up loads of close relations and food but do nothing
for neighbourly exchanges: it is a very lonely, suburban life. For me,
reinventing myself as a suburban mother involved learning a new
language of love. I don't think I did very well. Had I forgotten how
to love like an Australian woman?

I knew all of my neighbours in my London East End home. We
had a Portuguese nanny once, a young married woman named
Erica. She was our favourite. One night her husband was picking

her up on his motorbike. He was a courier. They reminded me so much of me when I was young and newlywed in London, trying to make our way in the world. I felt very protective of them. We were saying goodnight when this redneck guy in a car nearly swiped them off, stopping to make a racist remark based on the sticker on their motorbike, which lets everyone know which country you come from. He couldn't fling the insult and get away with it though. At that moment our neighbour from across the way, a Rastafarian, had pulled his van out and blocked his exit. He got out. He was big. More neighbours opened their doors and strolled out. All the kids from all the neighbouring houses, and the Rasta had a lot of kids, crowded around the car. They created a path for Erica and her man to escape on the bike. The poor racist twit was looking pretty scared. They let him go after a few more glares and comments about his sad ugly face. We never saw him drive down Glyn Road again, even though we knew he lived on the estate down the road.

Fast-forward to living in a huge family home with a swimming pool in beachside Australian suburbia. No one spoke to us. Was it the university car in a street full of plumbers? Our plumber in London, who'd been with us through too many home renovations, used to borrow my yoga videos, and talk all day about the state of the world. Here, in this world, our neighbours had written to the real estate complaining about how noisy we were, and that we didn't mow our lawns. One dewy dawn I was out walking with Scarlet and Hunter. It was before 6am and the world was quiet. But then one of the mothers hissed from behind her hose, *get away from my home with your retarded children*. Her sons used to ride their skateboards up our driveway and chuck rocks at the door. One neighbour used to throw things over his fence into the pool. Was it the English accents? After the ambulance had been more than once, and after we bought roof racks and surfboards, the vitriol stopped. No wonder I have written some rather uncomplimentary poems about suburbia, Australian style. For a long time, though, I couldn't read, let alone write. I don't tend to talk much when I am kissing. So I just shut up, and kissed my husband when he came home from cricket.

But life at this time was not all beaches and cricket and kissing.

QUESTIONS I HAVE ABOUT BEING SO DEPRESSED THAT I WENT MAD AND CAN I BLAME BEING ADDICTED TO LOVE?

When I was an undergraduate student at the University of NSW – I went there for the law school, it was a fabulous place, pity about forgetting to sit my exams – I was for a short time an English major. That is, before I realised the folly of sitting exams whilst high as a 747 on amphetamines. I had a look about me in those days that one boyfriend described as Laura Ashley on acid in go-go boots. This century, I sit in tutorials and listen to my students reading out their poems about ecstasy and all the different colours and names of drugs they took on the weekend and I think, *where has modesty gone? For a brisk walk to their dealer?* OK, so I'm an old fart. But who is going to pay for all their medical care when they hit middle age? No one cares. We just write poetry.

Anyway, before I failed English in third year and became a historian by default, I nevertheless had a lot of courses under my belt. One of them was on women and writing, a newish thing in those days. We had read a lot of Adrienne Rich. What a poet. At the time she ranked for me right up there with Radio Birdman and the Saints for lyrics (that was my 'day' job, music reviewing, no better job in the world in the 1980s than writing about Australian music, in Sydney, WOW). But it was feminist theory and criticism that this course concentrated on, so we were reading Rich's prose essays, *On Lies, Secrets and Silence.* Her list of things that keep women oppressed, I have never forgotten. The list included addiction to male love. Was addiction to depression in there? See, I have forgotten. Female horizontal hostility was there for sure (don't get me started). Unfortunately, I was addicted to love long before I read Rich.

I started keeping a diary during the time my first marriage was dying. I had been faithful to my husband the entire time we were together, more than 13 years; even after he left me my relationship with James was platonic for ages. No one believed this. I didn't bother disputing being cited in the divorce papers as a slut, a paramour, I just wanted to be divorced – what did the story they told to legalise it matter? The day I started writing this diary, I stopped crying myself to sleep over my dead baby. I decided to call it 'Diary of a Slut'.

AUTUMN 2001, LONDON.

We were oystered in a bench in Lincoln's Inn Fields, being shafted by sunlight. It was high morning, mid autumn, beautiful. Nowhere does parks better than central London, rimmed with their Regency glamour, or their Georgian promise. No one speaks better, in such a scene, than an English gentleman, contemplating leaving his wife. I had just spent the last 16 hours having the best sex of my life. Falling in love. It was hard to concentrate.

'You should!'

My mantra.

'Go back to her with an open heart!'

And now we were in a cathedral of light. The illumination hurt. With downcast eyes, I stroked his angora-trimmed wrist. I loved that jumper. The privilege of it all. His expensive clothes. His expensive accent. His expensive education. His aristocratic wife. His trust-fund children. One night together, and a few love letters of the century, was no real barter.

He gave me a cigarette. He lit it. I sucked slowly. He has begun his exit, I thought, it is too late.

'We went to the highlands this summer. I love it up there. We went with friends. Good friends. It was good. The house was right on the bay. Applecross is magic. I love that pub. We had dinner there every night. She didn't come out with us, ever. Blamed the baby. Well, she was only four months old. Every night, she insisted on the baby sleeping with us. In our bed. It was so high! Not even in between us, but on the outside of the bed. Jesus. There was a perfectly good cot in the room. And I was glad, you know, because I didn't want to have sex with her. But I was so worried about the baby falling out of the bed. And I asked her 50 fucking times to stop being so greedy and let the baby sleep in the cot, or in the middle of the bed. Just let the kid sleep. And that's what it's been like for 12 years. I am the cock, the sperm, the dildo, the host, the handsome bloody Englishman to piss the Scottish parents off. But I am not a father. Not a husband. She has never, ever, allowed me to parent the children. They. They belong to her. I lay awake, thinking about you know who and if I'd ever have the courage to be unfaithful, to fuck her, but I knew I never would, even though, well you know about my lovely wife and her boss. Then, sure enough, thud. She fell out of the bed, she did, that poor little baby. Then it was silent. There was no noise. And I knew then, in that moment before she cried, before I knew if the kid was dead or just hurt, that I hated her. That I was going to divorce her.'

I spent a little time thinking about the other woman he had been lusting after. Those Glasgow girls are some tough competition. One of them, a sociologist I think, had been after him for years. Jealousy wormed its way into the afternoon. The cigarette was making me feel sick. I didn't smoke.

'I have to go to work.'

'I have to go home to Edinburgh and leave my wife.'

You tell me: am I addicted to love? Anyway, that is what James did – he went home and left his wife and children. That was the endgame of our love, for soon, very soon, all that fresh love of ours turned to filth. It would always be thus: he will always be a man who left his wife and his daughter and his newborn baby for some slut in London. It seemed pretty fast to every single person around us, the speed with which James and I arranged our divorces and started building a different life, a life together. It was absolutely traumatic. It involved him walking away from an academic post in Glasgow that he'd held for over a decade, not knowing that it would take almost as long to secure another one. Want to look at our bank balance? And you simply cannot begin to cost what it has done to our children. We will be living through this forever. There is nothing for it but to keep fostering love in any way you can. To never give up. To love no matter what is said to you, about you, at you. There is, of course, the matter of our own love children, Scarlet and Hunter, and what we have visited upon them: thank you for the genes, Mum and Dad. To be loved is to be cursed is to be saved is to know love.

LOVE AND FEAR AND OTHER PATHOLOGICAL CONDITIONS

What does the sharing of all this really have to do with love, though? How much love do I expect to lose in the telling of this tale? Should I be more mindful? I decide to ask my first four loves – the children, James – if I should 'tell all'. Are you allowed to share secrets about people you love? They want to know what I would write. 'Well. I'll write what you let me.' Here is what they chose for me to say. They decided one story each would be enough.

Hunter
'Tell them I hit Scarlet's kangaroo. Tell them I want to be a superhero. Tell them I love my sisters.' When Hunter was three, we were at Aunty Barb's, she has a lot of kangaroos around her house. One was getting too close to Scarlet. So he walked over to it, jumped up

– it was much bigger than him – and punched it on the nose. He is fond of saying 'nobody messes with the Bradleys'. I pity his sister's boyfriends already. The kangaroo forgave him, I think it respected a primitive instinct.

Scarlet

'Tell them about me and Hunter having MCADD and how it happened and me nearly dying and the ambulance in London.' One night, Scarlet nearly died. She went in a blue light ambulance from Homerton to Great Ormond Street Hospital for Children. They saved her life. She has MCADD. Scarlet has been in a lot of ambulances.

Ulrike

'I can't choose a story. But I don't mind everyone in the world reading about me. Why would I? I'm *your* daughter. They don't know me. Like, *know* me.' Ulrike gave me her signature as proof she didn't mind. I could tell you a lot of stories about Ulrike. Her book is next.

James

James wanted to play too. But we were interrupted by the whisper of 'Mummy I'm still hungry', this after teeth had been cleaned and stories had been read. Our elder three children would be met with anything from '*tough*', '*next time you'll eat everything up*' to '*have a glass of milk, that will have to do*'. But you can't say that to Scarlet and Hunter. Say that to Scarlet and Hunter, they go to sleep, you go to sleep, they could die. We make crumpets and hot chocolate. More stories and toothpaste. Later, back to James: 'Tell them about me saving Hunter from being cannulated, from being put in intensive care when he was born.' They have a specific way of speaking to you, midwives. This one was sure I wasn't feeding Hunter enough, that he wasn't getting sufficient milk to stop him from possibly dying, so they wanted to give him formula. This was making me sad, but I knew, I knew full well, that MCADD babies are most likely to die within the first 24 hours. Everyone was very nervous, including the doctor who did his bloods. He was so nervous that he was shaking. He ran the test and it proved what he knew to be true. Hunter was going down. Off he went to get the relevant equipment. James, unconvinced by all this, snuck over to the machine and looked at the print-out. 'Insufficient Sample'. Hunter's stats had been misread and just as they were about to rush him through to intensive care, James made them stop. He made them all slow down. He did not want his son to suffer this. He did not want me to suffer it either. *Do it again. Run the bloods again.* You don't really boss medical people around like that. But everyone in the room took one look at James, and they did it again, and Hunter was fine. They left me alone, me and my baby boy, and we fed and slept and cuddled and fed all day and all night. We had to wait weeks for the official results for his MCADD-test to come back from the labs, confirming our fears. He was special, just like his sister.

Then there's me. I asked myself what I can tell you and what I can't and all I can say is if you're not bored yet, I have trunk loads of this stuff. Diaries, documents of terror that they are. Come on down. Before I light another bonfire, and fall in. It is not confessions that frighten me.

I am frightened of macadamia nuts because you have to hit them with a hammer to crack their shell, and I always hit my thumb. Or else start fires on cement, you have to hit them so bloody hard. They have lots of macadamia farms up on the north coast of NSW where I did my best growing up. Despite decades of acquaintance, I have never mastered this skill, the cracking of macadamia nuts, nor have I learnt to give in and buy them already shelled. I think it's time to surrender. And sharks. Sharks scare me more than I can say. I've seen too many in the surf to admire them as co-inhabitants of the ocean. They can have it.

I am frightened of sleeping. Sleep is not something I'm good at. Routines are there for the children, and they have a decent, beautiful, peaceful rhythm to them, there is no problem in our house about children and sleep, not now anyway. Sure, I used to have to feed them every two hours. Sure, they get up at 5am, Scarlet and Hunter, but they need to eat, they can't go any longer without food. Whenever I have even one night's fabulous sleep, I feel completely normal and madly, happily serene. I recall my best self. But this is rare. I have abandoned swapping tales of sleepless woe with other people. Everyone has them. At our staff meeting last week there were some funny and some sad stories about sleep and ageing and other things that keep you awake. I was silent. My sleeplessness inhabits another country, it has its own language and I cannot speak it to anyone. It is the language of a mother who sits just inside the door of her child's bedroom as they struggle with a common cold. Nothing to worry about – unless they have MCADD. I couldn't get her to eat more than a few mouthfuls all day and should I wake her up now for her emergency fluid and how far away from a heart attack will she be if I don't? Some doctors would say I am completely overreacting and others would say I should already have her in hospital, you can't take the risk. It is that divided, medical opinion, because the condition is so under-researched because it is so 'new'. Scarlet and Hunter are themselves research subjects. One day we will know more. Meanwhile, I don't sleep much.

I am frightened of offending people. I do not want to hurt anyone. Someone who read this book in an earlier draft said to me *why are you sparing them the boot?* My answer is that I don't talk to any of those people anymore, the ones who really hurt me, so I can't ask them if it's OK to tell their story. Hello! A girl has to have some ethics. Naturally, I can only tell you half the story. How frustrating for you, sorry, now you'll have to read my poems to read the ending. But not here, no, not in a memoir where you name names. Scarlet has very clear ideas about what I'm allowed to say about her, for example. I am not allowed to tell you, by any account, that she has a cute bottom. That's private, you see. There is an adult version of, or aversion to, the 'showing bottom' syndrome. I should know what it is, what constitutes transgression. Next time I see it I'll take a photo.

Love, I am not frightened of, not anymore, despite believing for too long that whomsoever I loved suffered. So for now, my biggest challenge is trying to make it up to Scarlet, recovering intimacy so that love can better flourish, and to stop thinking she is going to die, and continue believing she will live, that she will stay alive. There is only one way to recover intimacy. You have to spend time with each other. For the longest time, I was frightened to be alone with Scarlet. Now, we hang out. I am ashamed of every moment that I could and should have spent with her that I instead spent alone, trembling, whilst she was elsewhere. On Friday afternoons, I go to the school. I help out with maths tasks. I am useless at maths. It doesn't matter. I talk about her first, usually, every evening. Standing in the kitchen, after the youngest ones are asleep, sharing a glass of wine with my husband. I love to stand. I sit on my arse all day, standing is good. I love kitchens, too, mostly messy, warm ones, but standing around IKEA display 'life-simulation' kitchens also works for me, although you can't drink wine. Or have sex. You can stand around and write poetry though, in IKEA kitchens. Lucky for all of us that I usually don't. Hang out much in IKEA, writing poems, that is. How mad would that be! It's fun though. It's amazing how many arguments you can witness. James and I like to lie in the bedding section trying out the beds and kissing but the kids always jump on us. I love my kids more than I ever thought was possible for me, especially after spending so long in a big, blank space of despair.

The love of no man, my love for no man, has ever driven me insane. Not completely. Not independently. But, probably, it has, accumulatively. After all, it has not necessarily been sensible, healthy, nor a prosperous pursuit to chase a prototype of love and life that cemented itself to you, smash sudden, when you were still a teenager – that has decided a crazed path for me too often. The love for my children certainly has driven me a bit crazy, or rather my feelings of failure surrounding mothering. The loss of a child that you believed you cursed away, paediatric intensive care units and the fearing of further loss, that quivered love keeps you in a rough, homeless place. Without the love that began it all, the love that made those babies in the first place – who knows. Who knows. What if? What if it had been otherwise? I've left too much of my life to fate, and made too many decisions according to a roll of a dice. The outcomes have been uneven to say the least. To say the worst, if I were to believe my own poems, if you read them as confessionals rather than fiction, I would have no idea, honestly, why I'm still married, or why James would ever want to be married to me. In vino veritas, the ancient Greeks and Romans taught us, truth unfolds with the indulgence of wine. I've always argued instead that it was the intoxication of confessional writing that unbound all secrets, and made the most useful weaponry. These days, words and swords and dices and wine still inhabit my life, but their truths are less fundamental. I know less than ever. Because the dice has a seventh number. It is the one you can never see, it is the one that appears when the dice rolls off the table, and hits the wall, on the floor, rolling under the piano. That is the number, the place, where love for my husband and love for children collide, and it makes the piano shake. The grace of that shaking love, that is what shook my depression away.

Chapter 5

I have lived in an awful lot of places, and most of them have been genuinely splendid places to spend your life. I consider this extended, rambling encounter with difference – different homes, different landscapes, different peoples – to be a great blessing. But we all know how difficult moving can be, and how high it ranks in terms of its status as a major contributor to life stress. In my childhood, the regular moving to new towns was compulsory, because of the line of work my father was in, but as an adult, I have not changed this habit, despite now being more or less mistress of my own destiny. I even remain 'famous' with my friends for my endless interior decorating reshuffling – they cannot rely on finding even an armchair in the same place twice. As a writer, particularly the 'historian me', I have long been interested in exploring issues of place, belonging, and identity. As a self-confessed recovered (is it ever safe to say that?) depressive, I am also concerned that this endless wandering might not appear as glamorous as it once seemed, and instead be a masquerade for a sadder reality, that of the homeless little girl from the wrong side of the tracks. My fantasies include being able to return to the parental home and rustle around in the attic to find cherished relics from my childhood – I can whistle to the wind for that one.

The sad truth is when I was depressed, particularly closely after childbirth, I spent large chunks of my daily life wishing I were elsewhere – even if I was actually somewhere where I had recently thought I very much wanted to be. Wishing is the wrong way to describe what I was doing, actually. I would be breastfeeding, crying, for all I had lost. Instead of looking into my baby's eyes, my own glazed eyes would be picturing a scene, a place, a home that I could not return to. These losses were often real, but they were also often dramatised, or melodramatic and imagined. I would yearn, ferociously, to be released from the entrapment of wherever I was that I thought was killing me. 'Be here, now', was not part of my emotional vocabulary.

Very late in the therapeutic process, I was diagnosed by my psychiatrist as suffering from (amongst other things) chronic adjustment disorder. This refers to a psychological disturbance that develops in response to stress. In my case 'stresses' ranged from the 'severe personal crisis' kind including the abuse I had suffered in my workplace, to the 'major unexpected negative events' kind, witnessing in particular Scarlet's near death and repeated illnesses. Treatment is usually of the psychosocial kind (which I was already undergoing) and encouraging the development of behaviour modifications that enhance adaptation to changed circumstances. Basically, for me, this meant 'same old same old'. That is, I had to keep seeing the psychologist and be tutored in cognitive behavioural therapy. There is not much psychoanalysis in this kind of treatment, to say the least. Not much conversation, lots of instructions, often of the coals-to-Newcastle kind.

Meanwhile, I had more theories about place and displacement in my head from two decades of intense theoretical reading on the subject than any therapist involved in my care. I could, if they had asked, have told them what I needed to do, according to psychoanalytical theory, to improve my health. Such arrogance is particularly unbecoming, so I did what I usually did, and kept my mouth shut (this was with my psychologists – my psychiatrist would conduct long, intelligent conversations with me, at all times, but as I've said before, I did not get to see him until I was almost dead). While my psychologist was busy trying to tell me not to think negative thoughts, and take some exercise, I tuned out to this redundant prattle and sat there wondering about more important things – ask me something that matters, tell me something that I don't already know; that was my unrequited wish in too much of my therapy.

There I would sit, in these compulsory therapy sessions, silent and bored for the entire time, the whole time, silent. The silence was not an intentional rudeness, but my experience was that my therapists enjoyed talking more than I did. I would pray silently to myself for some kind of reprieve. Sometimes, trying to stay awake, I would ask questions, that were invariably met with perplexed silence. *Please, do you think there is an existential reason that might explain what has happened here, to me? What is your position on Derrida's notion of hospitality as being essentially anti-social and oppressive? Do you think aporia is a serious condition and how might it best be countered? Should I meditate on the landscape/deal with my past/ or join a local sand dune care club? Why am I writing solutions to my trauma in poetry that I can't enact in my real life?* Instead of listening to unforthcoming answers, I would sit there and think about how I recently read something about T S Eliot and his theory of the 'auditory imagination', and how a poem can communicate something real to us before we even understand it, and wondering if therapists can listen to patients like this, in this special kind of way. I would will them that special talent, as I sat, choking on my despair.

Meanwhile, I was writing my way to my own deeper understanding of what had happened to me, mostly through producing poetry. All other attempts at communication were inferior, to the point of obfuscation. How are you today, my therapist or doctor would ask. And I would reply like the well-brought-up girl that I was, politely, impersonally, correctly, not creating any burden on the listener – or so I hoped. And in my pocket, there would be a poem, its confessions burning huge holes in my thighs, full of grief and strivings to comprehend my failures to adjust, and my chronic shortcomings when it came to being, just being, where I am.

Alain de Botton argues in *The Architecture of Happiness* that we are different people in different places. He says that architecture itself can 'render vivid to us who we might ideally be' and that 'To speak of home in relation to a building is simply to recognise its harmony with our own prized internal song'. If it is true that we need home in a psychological sense because of our everlasting vulnerabilities, then we are all involved in the emotional purchase of place, be it a beach (not for sale) or a building (increasingly unaffordable to possess/do we anyway?). We choose home, we choose to love it, because in such a manner we affirm our identity. I believe this, firmly. I also believe that we can be completely different people in different places. So, for me, I began the lonely therapy of writing about place and the hunt for self, in what turned out to be my first collection of poems. It is no coincidence that the word 'exile' appeared in the title of that collection.

I'd come home from a therapy session, and my husband would ask, kindly, Did you have a good session today? I'd answer. Occasionally, he'd venture something more pointed like, You've been going a long time. Will you be finished soon, do you think? Or, Are you getting everything sorted out? I'd really try to answer. But I'd meet his kind, gentle inquiries, more often than not, with a constipated silence. Clearly, this was all my fault. It was my fault that I was sick, and my fault that therapy and drugs were not helping. Or so I believed at the time. So, if it was my fault, I was determined to figure out why on earth I was 'displaced', and to sort it out. This process, for me, began as ever with the philosophical, and historical. So, this part of the story is really describing how I tried to understand my biggest problem, through reading, and writing, and the benefits of that.

The problem was, I just wanted to go 'home'. It is the same kind of feeling as wanting your mummy when things go wrong. I wanted home, I wanted to be there, I wanted it to make me all right, to take care of me. But where was home? And was this desire a falsehood? Who am I to cause so much trouble about wanting to live somewhere else, when I was living with my loving family, in a part of the world that people consider paradise? The only thing I knew for sure, despite my trepidations, was that if I refused to explore these issues, then I would not get better. So, I began what I soon came to call my 'hunting flowers' therapy phase. I did not win myself very many friends, let me tell you. A discontented person who voices their discontent is nothing shy of shotgun blasting away at the good decisions all the people surrounding you have made. *What do you mean you don't think much of a suburban seaside Australia?* Boat rocker. *There is nothing wrong with the local primary school, kids have to learn to be tough in this day and age.* Loud mouth. *Why does every back yard have to have a swimming pool and every front yard a double-doored remote-controlled garage, and how do people actually hang out together?* Lonely lost depressed inadequate mother, too sick to go to work. *This is not how I remember Australia.* No choice. I had no choice but to dive down to the bottom of the rock pool and suck some sharp oysters.

SEARCHING FOR THE PEACE OF 'HOME'

When I left Australia for the first time – from Kingsford Smith International Airport, Sydney – I could not hear the words of farewell and love being spoken to me, so full was my head with the sounds that I believed I would never hear again: high tide at Bronte Beach, baby magpies, the gears of the 378 bus struggling to cope with Macpherson Street, climbing up from the Tasman Sea, 'the ditch' between Australia and New Zealand, to Bondi Junction. 'The worst farewells, strangely enough, were to places, rather than to people.' It was 1985. I had a degree in history, a one-way ticket to London, no backpack, but a suitcase full (stupidly) of Australian beer, T-shirts from independent Sydney rock bands to give away, and my collection of Patrick White novels. All a girl needs. I was sitting there, the first in our family ever to have travelled to Europe unless you counted men going to war, sipping champagne with my grandmother. Wishing myself away. I knew I would write to her, but it was her place, our place, the landscape that owned us that I would most miss.

Moulamein. Bega. Cobargo. Bermagui. Grenfell. Coffs Harbour. Lismore. Sydney. Ballina. London. Pforzheim. Munich. Berlin. Sydney. London. Sydney. Lennox Head. London. Edinburgh. London. Lennox Head. Melbourne. Inverloch. Melbourne. London London London where are you? The whole world wants a seachange (or 'seashortchange' as my mate Larry calls it), and I want to go back to Hackney. Hackney marshes, which they filled in with bricks once flung all over London from the bombings during the Second World War. Hackney, whose Homerton Hospital where two of my children were born is the only hospital in the UK to house a police station; so numerous are the knife wound victims. Gun mile Hackney. Desiring place, needing home, that home. Mad, clearly.

SCENE: A LUNCH DATE UPSTAIRS ON THE BALCONY OF A HIP RESTAURANT, OVERLOOKING THE PACIFIC OCEAN

CHARACTERS: AN AUNT/MOTHER, A DAUGHTER, A NIECE

SETTING: BYRON BAY (AUSTRALIAN SEACHANGE COSMOPOLIS), LAST YEAR, LATE SPRING

NIECE: Aunty, why do you move so much?

AUNT: Because it's fun, sweetheart.

NIECE: But we've run out of space for you in our address book. I think we need to buy a special one just for you.

AUNT:	What a sensible idea. What shall we order girls?
NIECE:	But surely it must be unsettling.
AUNT:	Hmm. I like the sound of this spicy vegetarian meatball thing. There's unsettling and there's unsettling. Who put this notion into your head missy? Do I look unsettled to you?

Aunt pulls a silly face. Niece laughs. Daughter rolls her eyes.

NIECE:	Well. Not you maybe. But, like. I've only been to one school. And. Well.
DAUGHTER:	And I've been to nine. And I'm 10 years old. Can we go surfing after lunch Mummy?
AUNT:	Good idea.
NIECE:	I never know where to send your Christmas presents.
DAUGHTER:	We live in Melbourne. Duh. [pause] You can't go surfing in Melbourne.
NIECE:	Or London.
AUNT:	Well. You'll never never know if you never never go.
DAUGHTER:	Mum. Shut up. Please?

Niece and niece's cousin, Daughter, are friends again. Aunt looks longingly at the wine list. Then wistfully at her watch. The day resumes. Sound of surf. Fade out.

Because my dad was a policeman, in NSW, like teachers, policemen have to go to where they're sent. Part of being promoted means moving to another station. We moved a lot. Me, I really liked this, although I do recall a rough patch following one move where I thought it might be a good idea to only eat food that I also liked to rub on my face. This was my young vegetarian self emerging, no doubt, but mostly it involved eating a lot of 'face-mask-qualifying' foods. I don't want to pretend it was all easy, but I am genuinely grateful for the diversity of experience in my early life, and for feeling that I really know the country Australia like I never otherwise would. It has probably allowed me whatever sensibilities I do possess as a writer.

However, it is received knowledge in psychoanalytical theory that frequent moving in childhood can contribute to adult malaise, ranging from melancholia to depression, and beyond. I'm not so sure a psychiatrist would agree that my early life acquisitions of 'sensibilities' and poetic relationships to landscape were worth it. For my brother, I think he was not so fond of change, and our frequent moving. He has certainly lived his adult life in a more steadfast way, and would never drag his kids all over the shop, like I have. I suppose there's nothing for it but to work harder to save up enough money for their future therapies. In the meantime, I live in Melbourne, feeling lost in my own country. I am raising my children as Victorians (not in the historical sense, but a geographic one) – if you do not think this is an act of migration greatly affronting this girl from New South Wales, please try singing all of the Australian Football League songs, team after team, at 'Footy Day' next year at our local Melbourne primary school.

What happens to people when they feel themselves to be away from their own idea of what home is? I believe your poetic genetic sensibilities mutate in a way that Darwin would understand, would classify. One day you find yourself in the wrong end of London Town and everywhere you look, from rotting Victorian mansions to the River Lea struggling to find its own clean pulse, it feels like home. The Australian bush, the pull of the Pacific Ocean, that light that can fry eggs, it all disappears from touch, sinks into lost memory. You realise that adoration and reverence had never had very much to do with your scrutiny of Australia. A policeman's daughter growing up in scrappy outback town gets to see a lot of ugly things in uncensored places, after all.

The Australian poet Peter Porter's 'Duetting with Dorothea' nails this feeling, that of not being in Wordsworthian concordance with place. Dorothea Mackellar's poem 'My country' was an anthemic experience for most school children, chanting our love for our 'wide brown land', our 'sunburnt country'. As a child, I missed the poem's insistence that we could never properly love another land like we loved Australia, but Porter explains the terror that lurked beneath the surface for all of those who failed Mackellar's ecopoetic breath test.

> But Dorothea's Country
> Did not seem mine when I
> First looked out of the window
> With costive childhood eye.
> Instead I saw a landscape
> Lit up by inner doubt
> And scarred by self-attrition,
> Not Barcoo Rot or drought.

So what happens when force of circumstances returns you to the place of sunken memories? Fact: one day my youngest daughter Scarlet nearly died. I could not think, while she was in a coma, where on earth I would bury her in London. Shortly after her recovery, circumstances saw our family emigrating back to one of my childhood haunts, Lennox Head, where my family lived, to raise the children in 'paradise'. To be free of London and all its ambulances with their blue light serenades. To be certain of the site of graveyards. I could find no poetry to underwrite this decision. All I had was a job offer at the local university, where, 25 years earlier, I had turned down a bonded teaching scholarship and run away to Sydney. To agree with Porter's sentiments became an irrelevancy. Or so I thought. Something was lit up by inner doubt, but it was not the landscape.

It was the French sociologist Emile Durkheim who introduced the concept of anomie, using it to describe a condition of deregulation in society, as he saw it. He suggested that when the rules of behaviour break down in society, then people no longer knew what they could expect from each other. He called this kind of confusion normlessness, and argued that it leads to deviant behaviour, either in the real or moral worlds. Criminality. Suicide. He was pretty concerned with the effects of social change, was Durkheim. As soon as social bonds cease to exist, life becomes impersonal, and therein the trouble begins. Is it true that we can't find our proper place in society without clear rules to guide us? Is it true that changing conditions and life adjustments lead to conflict? Durkheim surely argued that sudden change causes a sate of anomie. What else can one do when one feels like this, lost, unregulated, misplaced, except move again? Personal unrest is a curse; it is alienating and makes you feel uncertain about all decisions. This in turn erodes, for me at least, a sense of purpose that may have been fragile in the first place. If anomie can be thought to mean the state of being unable to find a psychological home in one's own society, then it is also responsible for its eternal re-creation. Who stays anywhere they don't feel at home? Well. I am. I do. Now. I am digging in. Trying to.

So much of my writing contradicts itself. I begin writing a love poem, only to find myself divorced by the end of it. Then making my husband breakfast in bed. He still likes my coffee, and me, I think, even though I write horrid poems about us. Is poetry trustworthy? Aporia is a Greek word that once meant a kind of puzzle, but when philosophers use it, it means something more akin to a paradox. Or, more, an *impasse*. Derrida was fond of discussing aporias, as his fans well know. He wrote a lot about how aporias and their paradoxes affect our notions of mourning, of giving, of hospitality. And of forgiving. Aporias have a logic to them, but not necessarily solutions. Derrida suggests, for example, that gifts are never really gifts, as they demand in their giving a reciprocation, even if it is only a humble thank you. And on hospitality – how can that be genuine when to be a host means to be a master, means to control your guests and if control is relinquished then so too is mastery, and if that is abandoned then you lose your home and can't be hospitable in the first place? On forgiveness, genuine forgiveness involves the impossible; that is, that we forgive the 'unforgivable'.

There's just no hope in some scenarios, is there, if you let Derridean logic castrate you? I'm convinced by these arguments, but what does one do with such information? Certainly, to be this philosophically confused, or combative, did not make me the easiest person to treat in therapy. Maybe it is completely unfair of me to have expected my therapists to have read these philosophers and sociologists and be acquainted with their theories concerning health and society, but that was my fantasy of what therapy would be like. Was I really expecting too much in wishing to debate these topics with the view to moving me further from my depressive illness towards health? I always turned to my writing, at least I could have an intelligent conversation with myself (if slightly unhinged!). I write this and think *who are you to be so bloody superior?* Who was I? A very sick woman. Lost. Making no connection to the therapeutic services on offer, for way too long.

FRIENDS AND THEIR POETIC IMPULSES: EVERYONE HAS SOMETHING TO SAY

Aporias. Anomie. Scarlet nearly died, and shortly afterwards, after one move too far, one too many, I too fell down, suffering a kind of nervous exhaustion that left me unable to fully care for three children, two under 2 years old who were both suffering from a debilitating genetic disorder. Does anyone else find it incredibly hard to choose a home, and in truth to trust the decisions we make on our children's behalf? We had chosen Australia, for their better health, but secretly I had no confidence in the sunshine – the power of place – to outweigh the displacement I felt from my own Australian people. To my shame I felt entirely apart from them. It may have been all those automatic double garage doors in contemporary seaside suburbia, and their ability to vacuum away congeniality. But here I am, here we are, facing all advantages and disadvantages for the greater good. Disembodied. Uncitizened. The rest of the world envying us our luck – or?

MAY 2006, LENNOX HEAD

Dear girlfriend,

Thanks for the pictures of your bubbies! They really are their own little people now. Seeing them makes me want to jump on a plane right away and come over and cuddle them. A coffee with you would also be nice. Some quick news, sorry, I have to go teach: we have accepted an offer on Glyn Rd, so goodbye London home. You know where my heart is, and what an ache this causes. But but but. The children are thriving and happy. James has just been offered a job, and we both feel safe enough about the kids' health to consider leaving them in childcare, if we can find the right person. Hunter is really a little English gentleman. He is the only longhaired, blonde surfie boy in Lennox who shakes hands with everyone and says 'How do you do?' and kisses ladies' hands and says 'Enchanted'. As you can see, James has been doing an excellent job while I've been at work teaching people how to write love poems about rainforests. God. Don't ask. Ulrike is surfing mad, and certainly looks the part. Scarlet is going to school in January, can you believe that? James is of course her favourite person in the world, having taken care of them for the last three years while I ran away to work and cried. Basket case. Great having the family around though. Our neighbours are truly atrocious, I don't know what has happened to this country, everyone is so greedy. They yell over the fence at us to shut up in the swimming pool! I think they just hate the pommy accents. Have to go, have to go, sorry. Write and tell me everything.

Lots of love
S

THE SAME DAY, LONDON

Darling S, my dear friend

I have just had a chance to read your email properly and have a few baby-free moments to reply, who knows maybe longer . . . all of the babies in bed asleep! How absolutely fabulous that you've sold your house, hooray! I'm sure it feels like you're cutting some ties but every-thing you've written adds up, the children, James's job, the life you've made for yourselves. What do I think? I think that it's nearly June here in London, it's perishingly cold, grey and miserable and we've had to turn the heating back on. I think that several times a day, by the time I've put on the children's wellingtons and coats, it's started raining too hard for us to go out and I have to try to explain again why we can't go to the park. I think that without the money to enjoy the cultural richness of London and without the long sunny days to enjoy the only things that are free, without the means to afford good schooling or the space and quality of air to allow your children's health to thrive, that it'd be a high price to pay for academic stimulation and the occasional company of some dear friends. That said obviously I would far rather you were just down the road available for coffee and cuddles but that would be selfish. It may seem hard sweetheart to be so far away from what you think you're missing but it's also easy to think that things would be better somewhere else. Perhaps you could view this as an experiment, stay still for a little while longer, feel the stillness, embrace the stability, nurture your body, your children's freedom, see how it feels ... London will always be here and you are not defined by your surroundings, merely living in them, benefiting from them. That's what I think for what it's worth ... I can hear someone crying upstairs. I love and miss you all and long to see you. But more than all that, I wish you some peace. Kiss all your beautiful family for me.

Huge love,
Bxxx

People have always got a lot to say to me about how lucky I am to live in Australia, and how they view my restlessness here as bad mannered. I have shed-loads of emails and letters telling me how privileged I am to live in Australia. But, these people don't even begin to know the grief of reconciliation, for example, and the sense of trespass that is your constant companion – mine, at least – as a white fella here. An Australian poet of some half a century's residence in London, someone who does understand, wrote me a postcard last year reminding me that when Melbourne turns to dust I can always come 'home'. Some people get it, some people don't.

I might be here, in Australia, but where is my head? London. How embarrassing. Obsession, aporia, whatever, it can't be good for your health. I'm thinking that maybe if I moved to New Zealand I might start writing love letters to Melbourne. Tomorrow, we're being visited by some family, down from Sydney. When I was still in primary school, I used to go to the beach with this cousin, along with his big brother, and my little brother. Being the eldest cousin, I was in charge. I think in reality this meant I was in charge of the sandwiches, as my boy cousins were the locals at this inner-city Sydney beach. We meandered our way down the hill from Henrietta Street, across a few, lazy, 1970s streets, finally making our way through the gully with its subtropical overhangs, to Bronte Beach.

Bronte Gully has many sites of Aboriginal significance that we were ignorant of in our childhoods.[1] We knew nothing, as kids. Nothing except that we were white (did we even know that?), and that migrants who loved to picnic in the gully, they didn't speak English. And we could swim better. And as far as surf life saving clubs go, Bronte Beach's was the oldest in the world. These things we knew.

Once we hit the sand that was it. God knows what we did, but we did it all day long, until starvation drove us home again, back up the hill to Mardie and Pop, our grandparents. Fish and chips from the shops up the road in Charing Cross, on mint green and dusty pink and powder yellow plates, sitting in the front garden, the salt already deep in our blood from all day in the ocean, and on our vinegared tongues forever. Our skin was tight, our noses peeling paper. We were as happy as rainbows in a mad summer storm.

Bronte Beach is a sacred place for many. Pop, my grandfather, was a Bronte 'splasher'. To own one of those gold towels with the royal blue splasher's insignia is a grand thing. Bronte has a sea pool, with lanes and diving platforms. That pool, it has seen some things. At low tide you can lap and lap. At high tide you can wait for the unforgiving waves to break over the rocks, and scream yourself wild as you let the ocean make you jump with it back into the unimaginable container of a pool, looking like an enormous Tupperware of promise, toying with you. Are the edges hard or soft? You go under. You hit the chalking bottom, and can't see through the churn of foam, but the suck and drag of the drama is gone before you surface. You get up, your seaweed-lead arms manage another poolside return, and you stand there looking out at the Tasman Sea. Where

1 Waverly Council. Bronte Park: 'A Pleasure resort at Nelson Bay'. www.waverley. nsw.gov.au/__data/assets/pdf_file/0005/8681/BronteParkAPleasureResort.pdf (accessed 15 March 2011).

are you? Here I am, it always says, just as you turn your back. The set repeats itself, tide in and tide out. It could be lunchtime, hours past, before you remember the boys. Or the surf proper. Or the lifeguards, and their whistles, and their Nazi concerns, way down the other end of the beach. It was, despite no adult supervision and the skin cancers that are forever surfacing in middle age, a safe, charmed, place.

I know people die at the beach. Sadly, I have seen this at Lennox Head. Two elderly British holidaymakers, they walked into the rip hand in hand, it was such a perfect day to die. And I've witnessed dozens of rescues over the years. My brother was recently on the scene at a shark attack. Surfers have never been the closest of friends with lifesavers, or shared the same moral codes, but may god bless Australian lifesavers. And now my children, religiously, on summer Sundays, know that their church is Nippers – the little people's version of the Surf Life Saving Association of Australia. It is, admittedly, paramilitary in nature. Sometimes it just doesn't pay to mess with the power of suburbia.

Before I'd ever give up on life, I'd set myself up as writer-in-residence with a little sign, in Bronte park, 'Writer willing to convert your Bronte stories into a book of Common Love'. Writing up all these prayers, these poems, would require a committed schedule of reincarnation. So to lay any special claim to the place would be mad, but by god I remain mad about Bronte. On the day that my eldest daughter Ulrike was born, I went swimming in the pool at Bronte. I had convinced myself that dedicated lap swimming would make the birth easier. My, how we fool ourselves, but I nevertheless had a lovely time with all the old biddies, the only other fools at the beach in late winter. A few days earlier, swimming, I had seen an octopus at the bottom of the pool. What if it lurched up and wrapped itself around my belly? I was huge, two weeks overdue. My last swim felt like communion – would I ever be able to chant to you like this again after you were born, this long hum of love, I wondered to my daughter? Would the opera of bubbles I blew for you hours before you were born be my last? I was booked in that afternoon for an induction, and induced you were. And tomorrow, the Sydney family who had surrounded you with love when you were born, who lived in Bronte, where we had moved from golden childhood to the honeycombed life of young adults at university, they were coming to Melbourne. May they own decent overcoats. No swimming outside in August in Melbourne. Ulrike and I went surfing last winter, our first down south, in respectable 'steamer' wetsuits, mind you, and it was the first time we had seen ourselves turn purple. It took a few days to find our pink selves again.

I was a child at Bronte. I lived a magical part of my adult life there too. I wrote my first book there, in a sun-flooded flat across from the beach. I remember myself then: and tomorrow, my Bronte cousin will arrive at our busy road in our shabby Melbourne suburb in a government car. He is a politician now, not much time for surfing these days. He and his family will be treated like royalty tomorrow, we are bereft of family down here at the bottom of a big island that one former prime minister called the arse-end of the world. Even ruder, Ava Gardner, starring in the movie of Neville Shute's dystopian novel, *On The Beach*, which was being filmed in Melbourne in 1959, famously said that there was no better place on earth to shoot a film about the end of the world. Well, you can take the girl out of Sydney, but . . . sorry, Melbourne. I will be upbeat about you, tomorrow, when they come. Please stop your raining.

Once, I was on the 378 bus from Bronte, where it began, quite early in the morning. Even the seagulls were quiet. Not like my travelling companion, a little old Jewish lady, who lived in the same block of flats as me, and had numbers tattooed on her arm. She was fond of my German husband, and approved of his motorbike ways, and us, and our marriage. We used to sit together, rocking and rolling up the hill towards the city proper. *Do you like Sydney my dear? Do you miss Europe? It isn't what it was when I was a girl, no. No. Well, of course it doesn't matter where you live. You know that. So long as you are with the one you love. That is all that matters. All that matters.* She had absolutely glorious hair, that lovely lady. She had a convincing style. I never asked where she was travelling to so early in the morning. But I have asked myself if she was right – is it people to whom we owe our greatest fidelities?

ON THE LACK OF GRACE, OR, HOW BEING STUPID AND STUBBORN CAN SLOW YOUR RECOVERY

Regret. Oh London, how I loved you. I will always be your slut. Sorry. Sorry to all my friends who write to me moaning of having to walk the children to school with their umbrellas being blown inside out. Sorry about having to turn the central heating on in the middle of summer. Sorry that your petrol is frightfully expensive. Sorry. Did you know it snowed in Victoria last Christmas? Sorry.

I have a habit of writing poems of apology to all the places I have loved, and left. I am so routinely unfaithful. Being in the right place can improve us, morally and spiritually. My resolve to be better, to be well, to 'identify' home soars as I age. Travel, and all the shedding and loss involved, has less appeal than ever. I have an even more unsavoury habit of writing poems about places I live that I am still developing a firm relationship with (the quest for love). So much of life reeks of that arranged marriage.

'Someone else's cool': prose poem for Amy

If you take this job, one day you'll be standing on the corner
of Plenty Road waiting for the 86 tram at an intersection
to kill all intersections, and you'll spy, waiting for the lights,
first in line, a plumber, 'Joe the Plumber', in his fluorescent
green ute, and sitting placidly next to him, moronic with
boredom, is his sad daughter. She has end-of-the-day pigtails
and a grubby-collared high school uniform and, really, could
do with some braces, bless her. *Why don't you just move
to Byron Bay and be done with it?* you will think, *If I was a
plumber that's what I'd do. Fix shit and surf.* You will think
this, you stupid woman, you who can't even afford a car
HOW CAN THE STUDENTS AFFORD SO MUCH PETROL? hence
the tram, and the wait, and you standing there thinking
this despite the fact that you know, you know, that all the
teenagers in Byron Bay wish they were in Sydney (note:
not Melbourne) or New York, anywhere but this suburban
dustball on a late sunsplit afternoon. The pollution. The
pollution. You will stand there, listening to Primal Scream
on your cold pink iPod remembering seeing them last time,
in Brighton, and forgetting that you once decided to write a
book about a deranged Gillespie groupie and the worship of
all things primordial, all the time praying that this green-uted
life will not be your daughter's. That she will be saved such
intersections. You will stand there twisting in the heat and
choking on everybody's urgent exiting, suddenly knowing
that leaving Stoke Newington Church Street N16 London and
St Mary's Church of England infants school where she was
the only white girl in her class was the dumbest-arsed thing
you ever did. To never again sit across from the school in Café
Vortex, chowing down to an egg and bacon sandwich and
the hum of your girlfriends also fresh from the school run,
their sweet talk like birdsong in a crystal vase, in between

breastfeeding and smiling at the singer from Cornershop
who is smoking and drinking coffee and writing lyrics and
laughing with his mate, to never again be so close to your
own shimmer, your true quickening, is irredeemable sin. Or, it
would be. If you take this job, that is. But, there is this, also,
to consider, that she may never know the lonely lusting for
honeyed Hackney evenings and the quicksand pull of long
summers in 50-foot gardens full of French wine and London's
naughtiest, your daughter, she may never credit it: all such
loss is someone else's cool. She may after all prefer Berlin.

Why so close to all this traffic?

In the mirror atop the hall table, in that crevice between frame and glass, there is a birthday invitation lodged, alongside a bill for the piano lessons, and, on top of them all, an old postcard from Geales, the fish restaurant in London's Notting Hill. It seems I have married into that family, Geale being my mother-in-law's family name. It has recently changed hands, again, that fine fishy bistro. It hasn't seen a Geale running the place in years. The houses around it are painted in pastels. The restaurant is in a suntrapped street in a magical part of the city. It serves many fine seafood dishes, but fish and chips is their business; so if their fish and chips is not among the best in town then they don't deserve their business. They do. When will it cease to be part of our pilgrimage, the lunch at Geales, whenever we hit London town? Stories can never be untold, but should it be necessary to forever behold? *You can't put your arms around a memory*, as Johnny Thunders said best.

I have never been back to Glyn Road, E5, despite years of tenancy that needed inspecting, and being in London as often as seven or more times in three or less years. In future, I plan to make similarly ripe, decent decisions. First though, whilst hunting wisdom down, it seems I have to spend more words retracing life than I ever did hours living it in the first place.

They do very good fish and chips in Port Melbourne. By the way.

CODAS BIG AND SMALL

NOVEMBER 2005, LONDON

Dear Diary

It has to be one of the most belligerent Novembers on record. Went to Katherine Gallagher's latest poetry collection launch, *After Kandinsky*, at the Menzies Centre. Beautiful poetry, like uninvented colours. As usual, there was a mob of interesting Australians there. Enchanting reading, with music. I felt horribly lonely. Ended up in gay bar in Soho, as you do. Finished interviewing most of the writers for the book (a literary history of Australian women writers living in London) all except a few of them insisting they are moving back to Australia soon. There goes another pig past the window. Convinced I don't know anything anymore. Can't wait to go home, go for a surf. I promise myself never to write a single poem about surfing. Or a research paper. About anything I love, lest it be sullied. Liar liar liar.

Back home in the subtropics, I wrote and wrote and wrote, poem after bloody poem, imagining every day I'd spent away from them, my family, and what transpired in my absence. My black absences. All of them. There were long, awful eulogies to all the streets I had lived in, and to that special shade of seduction that is a November London sky at 3pm. Then came the 'relief landscapes', terribly long, boring, unpublishable poems about rocks and sand and surf and their infinite possibilities. Writing, always, anthropomorphically. Like a child with an invisible friend, if I could not write myself into the landscape, if home was always slapping me or leaving me, then I would write it a speaking part and hope that it would choose me as its friendly director. What kind of citizenship is that?

Global mobility in this very transnational age remains costly, no matter the benefits. The moral code of respectable Western life peddles the belief that we should be faithful to our one love, and any deviation from that code is not normal. This same code also funds the idea that your loyalties should not be divided between countries, either, otherwise how can anyone properly answer the question 'Where do you come from?' Suffering from geographical schizophrenia for most of my adult life, it is no wonder that when the chips were really down, when I had to make the decision that none of us perhaps pay enough attention to – where would you bury your dead child? – my identity collapsed, and I could not recall who I really was.

Moving between continents, and assuming new cultures, insists on the attrition of skin, that which keeps us bound to ourselves. For me, part of that attrition was losing my sanity. I know that plenty of women who have never ventured out of the very suburb they were born in also suffer from postnatal depression; I am simply stating that if you were the kind of girl lucky enough to believe that she could do what she wanted to do and be who she wanted to be, and acted on that belief, when that dream crumbled, you had a much harder landing than many others to cope with. Documenting such attrition, such side-effects, such costs, became for me the very core business of poetry. No one else seemed to want to listen to the conversation.

Not many people, from lonely, needy, ageing parents to confused children to told-you-so psychiatrists, respect your decisions to choose a nomadic life. As I, too, begin to waver in my steadfast respect for all these enactments of desire, I can only revisit the sites – psychologically – and hope that what memory offers is worth it. This is perhaps the last landscape of refuge for the writer seeking sanity, that relationship with memory. It has its own special geographies, its own responsibilities. Theory and history, where the poetics of place are concerned, can only offer limited consolations. As much as they might help one to understand their place in the world, memory is sometimes a woman's better friend, no matter how haunted a country that may be. Illness, in my case, certainly did something peculiar to landscape – you are there, inhabiting it, but you are also not: '[H]ow astonishing, when the lights of health go down, the undiscovered countries that are then disclosed', Virginia Woolf wrote. She also insisted that our need for poets is paramount when contemplating life from the perspective of anyone who has done living out their embryo lives: 'We need the poets to imagine for us. The duty of Heaven-making should be attached to the office of Poet Laureate.'[22] Perhaps Woolf is right, that it is so essential a task that it is best left to poets, this urgent need to know our destined 'country'. I would add that the quest to know our lost homes (our past) is similarly vital. For me, thinking about the past, and where I belonged, was vital to my recovery. Sure, take the drugs if you can, take any therapy that works, but think about the future as well, and don't be frightened to imaginatively engage with the past: I spent as much energy trying to stay standing up as I did planning not to fall over again. Keep your fingers crossed, please.

---

2   Woolf, Virginia. *Selected Essays*. Oxford: Oxford University Press; 2008. 101, 107.

Some people stay where they are born, some people head for the closest metaphorical or real airport, walking through the shadows of early dawns trying to conceal their own sad departures. The place I want to know most is trapped in the past, a past lived in real place and time. In London. And later, at the beach, in Australia. I know this to be true because I have seen the photographs, I am there, confined, in silence and light. My children were there, but I was not. One doctor called this 'absence from home/from self' postnatal depression. Another called it chronic adjustment disorder. I just call it poetry, on its usual hunt, for the smell of home.

Chapter 6

The true shape of a pear

I once read, in one huge insomniac gulp, a fabulous book written by an ex-playboy centrefold model (now suburban mother of four) about how to get your groove back post-childbirth. It made me laugh, and gave the odd piece of excellent advice, but I was nevertheless fairly sceptical about some of its more dubious recommendations. For example, about sex, where the main advice was not only to just do it, but also to fake complete enjoyment of it. The rationale was not only that marital relations were worth preserving through this restoration period, but that in the act of pretending you might be surprised how a fake moan can transmute into actual and real-felt pleasure. For the record (but by no means as a recommendation – more on that later) I had resumed sexual relations with the husband of my two youngest children as soon as coming home from hospital. While I was happy that things were 'business as usual' (and what was I really frightened of if it wasn't, I wonder?), after reading this book I thought, OK, I'll make an even bigger effort, I'll pretend to not just enjoy the closeness and the intimacy (which was true) but also the eroticism of sex. I pretended and I pretended and – it worked. This trickery of pretence soon became a wider metaphor for my life. As a metaphor it was fine, but in practice it became my downfall.

With only two weeks' paid maternity leave, an unemployed husband, and a pressing financial need to go back to work, I did my best to wean poor baby Hunter, only just diagnosed with MCADD. This also involved leaving Scarlet, freshly home from hospital and still recovering, with a new nanny. What was I thinking? The thing I hated most, still hate, about postnatal depression is how it turned me into a robot, how it robbed me of sense, how it stole me from my children. It is so insidious I thought I was normal, making normal decisions, yet they were based on a rationale that had been bankrupted by depression. James had an offer of a contract academic research position, but we were both too frightened to leave Scarlet alone for long, so his engagement with his workplace was sorely tested, as was mine. Scarlet was still recovering from her coma, and had not yet managed to walk, despite the fact that she had been standing before she fell ill. Someone had to go to work or we wouldn't be able to pay the mortgage. Someone had to watch the nanny watching the babies. You can't leave MCADD babies with a nanny. Not the kind of nanny that we could afford. I went back to work. They hadn't even sent me flowers when Hunter was born. They were fairly pissed off that they hadn't noticed I was pregnant when I was offered the job, and had never managed to recover their grace. For these kind of people, for this kind of job, I left my children. I thought I was fighting for the future, but all I was doing was squandering my life, and driving myself into deeper depression. Small wonder that a few months later I ended up singing with the grasses in Giraween, and enjoying a nervous breakdown. Hallucinations, though, can be a way of processing reality. I processed, and processed, and I guess that is what you are now reading – the reality that resulted.

It might be counter-intuitive, but I thought at the time that work, that 'keep-on-keeping-on' conduct would not only keep my family safe, housed and fed, but also that if I stayed away from the things that frightened me most – my children – then this would be best for all concerned. And when friends came around in London, we were all too busy admiring our newly landscaped garden to talk about much else. We all had new babies, that summer, me and my closest friends, or very young children. We were all exhausted – my friends ran their own thriving, demanding businesses, or were professors running large grant research projects, or were mounting exhibitions, or were full-time mums with husbands who were jetting around the world and being important and never there, or out-of-work actresses with the daily grind of auditions and no one to babysit the kids, and writers who couldn't finish their books because they were working too many shifts at the pub. Oh yeah. And parents. There was a lot of laughter and barbecues and fun, and an enormously joyous christening and brunch that lasted all day, with godparents coming from as far away as the USA. But after everyone else had left, had gone to bed, had finished sharing their own stories of woe and decided their husbands were worth going home to after all, there was just me. And the dark hound. He did not shut up, that dog, though I managed to banish him every time I fed Hunter, which was a lot. Hunter slept in our room, in a Moses basket beside me. He was my lifeline. I had to stay awake all night long to smell him, because in the morning I would desert him again. All of them.

Many advices about depression insist that you should not be ashamed about it, that you should be 'out' about it, that it is a time in life when you deserve to put yourself first, and that doing so is essential to your recovery. With no disrespect to medical expertise or to those for whose lives have been saved by this strategy, for me this approach is debased. There is a fine line between stupid denial (my own history) and sensible acceptance that yes, you might be sick, but *hello*, there are other people in your world who need you more than you need yourself. I did not tread this line successfully, but I still insist that thinking of others and not just myself saved me, as well as caused me some suffering. The suffering was minor, compared to the salvation. My husband still plays cricket. I am extraordinarily grateful for this for many reasons, not least of which is that he is a healthy role model for his young son. When Hunter graduates high school his parents will be 60 plus. We need to do what we need to do. Sure, Saturdays in Melbourne can be a drag, but the kids have their own kind of kid fun and I get to write nasty poems about cricket. It's all good, it's just life. Me and my depression are not the only people in the house that need attention.

Shortly after Hunter was born Scarlet ended up, as dramatically and rapidly as usual, in hospital. One of Hunter's godmothers was living with us at the time – our house was large, shambolic and run down, set in a rough part of town, but always full of beautiful people – and my Mum was over from Australia. Thank god. We had been let down at the last minute by James's Mum who said she couldn't come down to mind Ulrike and Scarlet for the birth after all. No idea why, but I knew she was on antidepressants. Mum had arrived the day I was to be induced – all three babies induced so very late, it has always grieved me that I couldn't manage this biological feat on my own. But on that night, James was in hospital with Scarlet, Eilish was busy worrying about her Spanish lover, and Mum was roundly yelling at Ulrike, for nothing. I was breast-feeding. I put Hunter to sleep, went downstairs, put Ulrike to bed, phoned the hospital and could not find out if Scarlet was out of danger. I then yelled at my poor guests saying that I felt rather put upon and I would appreciate it if they would leave. Immediately. Please. Perhaps it was a tantrum. I certainly said that I felt no one was giving me any space for how rotten I felt. 'What do you mean how rotten you feel?', screamed Mum. 'I mean with this depression. I'm so depressed.' And embarrassed. I felt hotly ashamed. 'You're depressed! I'm the one who's depressed! With all this to put up with! I'm the one on medication!' I looked at my darling mother. I knew in my blood all that she had suffered in her life. I put her to bed. She was sad for weeks, until she went home. I ruined her holiday. These women, our mothers, they are our elders. If they can't be there for you, they have their own good reasons. When it comes down to it, I am not one to hold it against them. As for Eilish, she cleaned up the kitchen and picked herbs from the garden and made supper. Both of us hoped James and Scarlet would be home soon.

The other reason why I am no fan of the privileging of 'Those who are depressed' in families is that – aside from the fact that there is often more than one person to service – I truly believe that melancholia is both a gift and a curse, and it is ultimately up to each individual to forge their own relationship with this integral part of themselves. Help and support in doing this is good, sure. No matter how old they are. I don't advocate a mindless pop-psychology solution of positive thinking, either. I just find the whole contemporary concept of 'all entitlement, no responsibility' completely vile. Each to their own. Each to their very, very own, with my respect.

FUMBLING AT MYSELF – WRITING, HAPPENINGS OF THE HAND, AND RECOVERY

Part of trying to get my groove back, beyond the bedroom, involved a lot of prescription drugs. One of the reasons I could not and would not continue with them is that while they all did different things to me, they had one thing in common: a robber-gene for creativity.

On one particularly speedy number, I did manage to stomp out an article that is so very 'out there' that it has quite sensibly never been accepted for publication.

When I was first ill following the accusation of plagiarism, I opened the newspaper one morning and found I could not read it. Later, on my own, I put all my pens and papers away, after trying to write an email and failing and having already packed up the laptop. Shaking, embarrassed, I went across to the beach, hoping no one would see me. I went for a long walk. It was if, I thought, halfway to Broken Head, that it was words themselves who had betrayed me, and writing that had accused me. They had, and not the student, not my colleagues (such scrupulous unionists!), not the lawyers, not the press. Words had betrayed me, words became my enemy.

This distrust soon extended to speech. I was fluent, mechanically, for the hour or so of therapy each week, and the consult with my GP, but silent otherwise. I like to talk. I stopped talking. I used to sit drinking on the balcony each night and talking to my husband. I stopped drinking altogether. Talking about what had happened seemed to lend it a life I resented. I became silence. Silence became me.

One of the reasons I believe that 'talking' as therapy did not help me, was because I resisted it. My participation in therapy was false. This is not a condemnation of the therapists/psychologists and others, who were all excellent in their own ways, but it is instead a reflection on me as a patient, and my therapists' inability to under-stand that my most defining feature as a person at that time, for me, was that I was a writer. Who couldn't write. Who had been accused of being a fake.

My therapy was compulsory and paid for by the insurance com-pany because of the fact that I had suffered a psychological injury in the workplace. That injury was the false accusation of plagiarism. Ostensibly, because someone had called me a liar, I had suffered a nervous breakdown (I am feeling very lame writing this story down: sticks and stones!). But as we know, and my last psych had the smarts to figure out, that injury was just one of those camel-collapsing straws. The camel had in fact been eating far too much black dog food for far too long.

When it first happened, that workplace injury, I too was less aware of this than I might have been, so it is no surprise that my therapists couldn't find out what I was really upset about. I couldn't admit it to myself. And, later, when I started writing out my grief in the poems, I could not immediately recognise or admit this 'true self' as mine. If they wanted to know about me they could bloody well ask the right questions. God, I was bored. I spoke fluently when trapped in therapists' rooms. I was talking my way out of there. It has long been part of my knowledge base that the sooner you give them what they want the quicker they'll leave you alone.

I was never interested in what the therapists said, because I knew as a writer they were failing characters, not being privy to 'protagonist' me. The narrative was nonsense, a poor story with an unfaithful structure. James gave up asking me how it had been when I arrived home. 'Boring', was always my answer. That is what a long-sustained lie always is in the end – boring. I respect and regret that my therapists may take offence to this supposition that they did not know I was performing, for I may be wrong, and if so please forgive me. However, one of the most revealing things said to me during all this medicalisation was by the psychiatrist appointed by the medical insurer, who was an observer, periodically assessing my needs, progress, and care: making sure that I was indeed eligible – that is, injured and participating in appropriate recovery programmes. Otherwise, all treatment and indeed my pay packet would cease. He also had veto on whether I was well enough to go back to work – couldn't risk a re-injury! This psychiatrist was very dismissive of the psychological treatment I had been receiving stating that in his opinion I was too interesting a person, and therefore too challenging, for the therapeutic relationship to be trouble-free: 'They are more likely to want to be your friend than your medical professional'. Hmmm. What are you meant to do with information like that, casually offered as you are leaving a consultation?

This same psychiatrist was the one who stopped my acupuncture treatments, which was in my opinion the only treatment of any benefit whatsoever. My acupuncturist, Jackie, was the one who helped me find sleep, who talked to me on a metaphysical level about the ghosts of depression according to Chinese medicine, who I ran my treatment options by: 'They want to send me to a private loony bin'. Jackie shared my shock and outrage at the suggestion of ECT, she knew that my life had had enough brutality for the moment. She knew more about my health and my walking towards it than anyone. I did not perform with her. She was the only one I told what I was writing about, on each visit. She was the only one who asked. She was sincerely interested in me as a creative artist, and her treatment of me took this into account. How, I know not. Are there special acupuncture points for neurotic writers?

If this account of me as a writer was being taken by other therapists, they never let me know. But back to the psychiatrist who put a stop to all that acupuncture 'quackery'. He said to me that the problem I was experiencing in my recovery was that I needed to see someone who was a good deal smarter than me, and that that was not happening. It did happen, eventually; we know this story has a happy ending. But back then, such an immodest thought had not occurred to me. He was right. He had to be, he had a vested interest in getting me off his books, in keeping me away from timewasters.

When I started again with words, poetry was the first language with which I could speak. I am party to Julia Darling's insistence that poetry comes to us when we most need it. It has that facility. But, at the same time, I hope that I never fully come to comprehend what that facility is. Writing is such a core compulsion, and contains such a complete history of pleasure, that to understand the process would be to nail a soul's tail to the garage floor and watch it flail and die. I think I have to get a different teaching gig.

My point here is to suggest that writers have – perhaps like other artists, but I can't speak for anyone, really, except me . . . OK – I have interior worlds that are warehouses of emotional and intellectual sorcery. And if you are trying to understand someone, understand them well enough to help them, and if they have a psychiatric disorder, then to leave that warehouse closed, unexplored, to not take account of its contents and how they nurture the owner, then to do this is probably a wanton act of neglect. But, I'm no doctor. Hell, it was boring. How interesting all that talk might have been. 'Why do you write?' Such a question can kill a dinner party but for me and my therapists I think it would have been a conversation worth having. It could have salvaged any one of the medical and therapeutic relationships I was in which, instead, beached themselves, one after another.

My second form of talk, when I got my pens out again, was my journal. The 'Big bad mad journal', as I call it, is an old beast. It seems to have a thousand pages in it. Often, it is not written in for a year or more, only to be filled with summative insertions, corralling up, say, a divorce or an intercontinental move that happened some time ago. My journal is not my confidante, nor my dumpster. It is a sparingly used, impressionistic canvas. Looking back at my journal over the worst period of my illness has allowed some insight. When I was at my clinical worst, I could write nothing but poetry. When my health improved, and my rationality, I wrote reflectively. I wrote, dragging myself up back into the real world, genre by genre. As soon I could write a lecture again, the very next day I went back to work.

MARCH 2005

Dear Diary

I'm about to go and give a lecture and it has just occurred to me why I
do what I do. Why I've always wanted to do it. It's a heroin-factor thing,
that hit that comes when a piece of writing perfectly calibrates. It is
exactly the same kind of hit I felt when I wrote my first history essay
with footnotes and a rhetorical argument. On the Persian Wars. Thank
you Mrs Keats. Except now, after the high, I feel bad. Did I really write
that? You have the faded critical acumen of a depressive. Perhaps it is
all rubbish. Too late. I have to go. Ordinary me must go and excite 130
students. Maybe I'll read them a poem instead.

Since that time, I have paid better attention to what I write, and
when. Novels simmer. On long walks their plot and characters
accompany me. Academic papers and research and lectures are
written with both journalistic enthusiasm and scholastic habit, hard
yakka, like walking through cane fields, excited by green ghosts of
cane whispering by your side with their sweet promise, but hot and
frightened of snakes, you cannot deviate from the process of thinking, accounting, explaining, defending, supposing, and postulating,
plotting your certain way through unknown fields. But poetry. Oh
poetry. It is like the baby's cry at 4am, never to be refused. When I
am writing poetry I cannot possibly answer the phone or turn off
the sprinkler or even remember the running bath until I have made
sense of these images that have visited me. My baths are forever
flooding the house. It is a very bad thing to be a writer in Australia
in the middle of a world-class record-breaking drought.

Maybe the real reason I never told my therapist – until the last
psychiatrist – anything of import is because I do not think that such
horror has any rightful place in spoken conversation. Speaking
is not the right medium; a speaker and a listener are not the best
vessels for such exchanges. That is why poetry exists, to speak the
unspeakable. Some poems I can never read out loud; that is their
currency, screaming silence.

As I keep saying, there is life beyond poetry, and the real groove
that I needed to find, to get well, was not just about me or writing.
It was about where my children were, and what sand dune they
were hiding in. Did they remember me and love me or was I as lost
to them as I felt to me? They couldn't read my poems to know how
much I loved and feared for them. I put them to bed each night and

kissed them but I had no idea what cereal they ate, even though I had fed them that very morning and would feed them the next. It was time to start some plain speaking.

WEETABIX AS DOMESTIC CEMENT AND OTHER SUCH WORLD VIEWS

What kind of social and emotional competence can I expect my children to have when they have had such a depressed mother parenting them? I know that clinical studies tell us there is no set answer, and that it also depends on the marital status and the health of the marriage and the mental health of the father. Peer relationships also matter. Lots of things matter.

When Scarlet was under the care of GOSH in London, they were also concerned to measure her psychological and neurological development, she having been in a coma as a result of the MCADD crisis. She was attending the Wolfson Institute, where they were doing just that, where she was to have that specialised care and attention all her young life. There is no such opportunity in Australia, and we have been through three state systems trying to replicate it. Such care is a pipe-dream. Nothing, nothing makes me want to go back to London more than sitting in the Royal Children's Hospital, Melbourne. Sorry.

I believe that a child's relationship with their mother and the larger world is mediated by how close you are, mother and child, in the first 18 months of life. I believe that I failed miserably with all my children, but most of all Scarlet, to secure a proper relationship. I know that attachment to children is affected by all kind of difficulties, and that I certainly had some to contend with. Will someone tell me what to do with this grief? But wait first, please, while I tend to the enduring effects on the psychological development of my children, accrued by exposing my babies to my maternal depression. How many times did my lapses in self-regulation and the revelations of what should probably have remained private cause them damage? How often have they been exposed to disturbances in their environment, how many chances have been afforded them to experience, absorb and replicate my own dysfunctional emotions and behaviours?

Lots of things contribute to the deleterious effect of maternal postnatal depression. One factor would be, in my world view, that getting depressed about all the damage you have done is nothing but counterproductive. I try my best to protect them from me. I once asked Ulrike's father to have her for the summer holidays just after Hunter was born. I knew what was coming. He said no. He went to Thailand. Don't talk to me about bad behaviour.

But what if our 'bad behaviour' is really not our responsibility, or fault? What if your genes own you? Plenty of studies suggest biological determinants for depression. OK. I surrender. No. I can't. I need to save that white flag for another battle. Knowing that my two littlest ones could die if they ever, for example, drank so much that they vomited. It is sobering. Confronting. Terrifying. Hell, it might even prove to be an effective parental threat in the not-too-distant future. There are some things whose pathological veracity shouts, 'hello, are you listening'?

Sunday morning. It is raining. It is a winter movie morning. We watch a DVD together cuddled up on the sofa, Scarlet and Hunter and me. Afterwards, following second breakfast at 8am, they play and I write. Their game is about the beach, and I stop writing and look at MCADD parent support sites online for the first time in years. They seem different. On the family stories pages, there are the same memorials and always poetry, but now there are more stories like Scarlet's – 'there go we but for the grace of god' stories.

Maybe this has a lot to do with parent and medical advocacy in recent years concerning supplemental screening for disorders, MCADD among them. This costs as little as $25, and up to $95 dollars in the US from what I could gather, but it is not only a question of economics – and how many people don't have the spare money for extra tests? – it is an educational issue. Most parents-to-be aren't even aware of the value let alone the dire necessity for 'supplemental' screening. The family of one poor boy who didn't make it have since been responsible for ensuring that their local state representatives in Mississippi passed a bill making it law for doctors at least to have to make parents aware of these additional tests. The bill was titled, 'Ben's Bill', after their son. In Australia things are changing all the time, and vary from state to state. In Victoria where we live, supplemental screening has been in place for 30 years. The hospital of birth is responsible for offering the newborn screening tests, and if the parents refuse they are meant to be referred to Genetic Health for urgent discussion. If the answer remains 'no', they have to sign a written statement saying they understand the health risk involved.

Scarlet and Hunter were not born here.

They come into the study. *Why are you crying, Mummy?* We look at the website together, and all the photos of the little MCADD children, just like them, who have gone to heaven. And some who had just made it, like Scarlet. We read all of their stories. Scarlet and Hunter want to know if my book about them will have their photos in it. They'd like that. They know I write poems about them, they ask to hear them, but this is different. They have never seen a picture or met anyone else who is like them, who has MCADD.

We decide to have some morning tea, and do some cooking together for a special Sunday lunch. Food is important in our home. Eating on rainy days is extra nice. That night, at supper time, they are extraordinarily naughty, and are sent to bed without dessert, or a story. Hunter is contrite. Scarlet storms out, five minutes later, *What do you think you're doing, trying to kill me! I'm still hungry.* Hostages, we are all hostages.

EVERY DAY I GO TO WORK AND MY BABIES HAVE MCADD, I AM A BAD MOTHER

Each semester our timetable changes. James and I never know what our hours will be in the long term. Despite universities and their claims to be child-friendly workplaces, teaching hours run from 8am to 6pm, often with longer evening obligations for postgraduates, and good luck to you if you can manage to rectify a timetabling obscenity – how can one teach until 6 when the kindergarten shuts at 6 and is a 45-minute drive away? – against the odds. Isolated in Melbourne, with no family or additional support, we rely on what is known as before- and after-school care. When Scarlet started school last year, this is the right word to describe the process of trying to educate the school community about MCADD: [please insert adjectival expletive of choice] nightmare. There were meetings with the principal. Her teacher. With the after-hours team, who as it turned out, were the only ones to pay proper attention. We provided information packs from the hospital, we provided medical records. We even, against our better judgement because it is rude to tell people how to do their job, suggested to her teacher that she might want to try giving Scarlet a snack instead of punishing her with the naughty-girl-who-won't-pay-proper-attention mat. Things got uglier. Day after day Scarlet was coming home with a full lunch box. Day after day we'd front up to the office and explain that it was terribly dangerous for her not to eat regularly. Not to mention make it hard for her to be robust enough to learn, to behave, to socialise. *Yes. Of course. We're onto it.* Like hell they were. It took Scarlet having a serious collapse and the ambulance being called whilst she was in aftercare for a 'review of her situation' to happen, and for an appropriate management plan to be instituted. Now things are excellent. Her teacher keeps a daily food diary and feeds her regularly. Scarlet has had to repeat a year, sure. She could have died then, on that afternoon not so long ago.

She didn't die because Ben, my favourite of the after-school care team, saw her going under and took her in his arms and fed her, and Scarlet let him because they liked each other, they had a good relationship. I adore him of course. It is beyond that though – he probably saved her life. Me. I was teaching an undergraduate class of first year students, none of whom had even bothered to read that week's text under discussion. I hate myself. Are my students worth placing my children at risk for?

'How I mark them'

It begins with diligent and courteous commentary,
and corrections, 'a promising piece', but after the
strict washboard of boredom is duty-fulfilled, and
work has become, again, Saturday, Saturday night,
Sunday morning essay marking, the only thing that
is fine is the wine, and the memory of smart sex that
morning as Dora explored the world.

You're wondering what it would have been like for
Sylvia, undead, old, widowed now, reading Ovid
on Sunday mornings in Primrose Hill. You look
down at your student's work and wish they
had written you a river. You almost write
'Try accountancy', but don't. Your children are at
the beach, without you. They may be hungry.

Suddenly, the purchase of one said café
at Fish Creek, 'for sale', seems like a retreat
that even St Crispin would have sanctioned.

As much as I fantasise about leaving work, it is not going to happen. We are broke, I am embarrassed to say, and cannot afford to live on one wage. Doing so for all those years when James was primary carer for the children was what has made us this broke, used up all our resources. We don't lament this, except for the anxiety we feel about not being in a better position to provide long term for our children, which is also one of the reasons why we are at work now. But at what risk? How vulnerable are they?

I read so much medical literature and it can be confusing. It is a new field. The first MCADD patient was only identified in 1982. When things are happening the children present with a constellation of features. We know it begins with hypoglycaemia and lethargy. We have seen it move beyond this to seizure and coma. Cardiac arrest and death are on the same calling card. That's the vulnerability stakes. Vigilance is funded by our hope that we will avert any such fatality. Our attentions are better directed towards monitoring long-term outcomes of not dying: developmental and behavioural difficulties, ADD, cerebral palsy, mental retardation, than worrying about the children dying. Studies of the developmental, behavioural and neurological disabilities as long-term outcomes of MCADD are, understandably, only just beginning to surface. I could tell them some stories.

TOUGH LOVE AND OTHER DRUGS OF RECOVERY

The children are not home. They have gone to the footy with daddy. At half time at Princes Park the kids are allowed onto the oval for a kick. Australian football is a good thing. Have I told you this about the children? They are huge for their age; both Scarlet and Hunter are at the top of the growth charts. Scarlet is not so robust, and goes down quickly when ill, but when well they have enough vitality to reanimate the dead. Ulrike has taught them both to ride a surfboard. Hunter was so young when he started that people used to stop and stare in wonder. They are not frightened of large surf or being dumped or footballs in the face, or terribly much really. Once at the children's hospital in Sydney, having their bloods done with a room full of other unfortunates, they were the only two kids not crying. One and all were impressed by their laissez-faire attitude to medicalisation and pain. Scarlet wants to be a rock star (good idea, no one will notice she's weird or at least it can be a worthwhile professional credential) and Hunter wants to be a superhero and to go to superhero high school and superhero university where daddy teaches and play superhero football where they jump really high. He seems to have the physical goods and the right psychology, even if he did spend the first four years of his life wearing skirts.

They are not home and I am frightened that they will have an accident and need surgery and will die. No one will perform surgery on an MCADD kid unless the holy trilogy of surgeon, anaesthetist and metabolic consultant are present. Not so easy to muster as you might think. It took us 18 months to get Hunter's teeth fixed. I am being silly. I am worrying about nothing. Of course if they have an accident they will find the right people and not fast him to death. But what if James dies in the accident and Ulrike forgets (she would not, ever) and no one can tell the ambos that the kids have MCADD – then they will for sure die in surgery, fasting too long. All shocks and accidents enhance their metabolic crisis, their need for energy is genetically denied them thanks to that absent enzyme. I need a Valium. I should have gone to the footy. I need to get a grip and treat them as normally as possible.

Sometimes, it is true, you have to be cruel to be kind. I smacked Hunter's bottom once, when he needed sleep and he was fighting it tooth and nail, and running outside and jumping in the pool in his pyjamas, and being an all-round rotter, and it worked. I cuddled him straight afterwards and said 'I'm sorry I had to smack your bottom, I love you, I want sleep to be yours', and we kissed and made up and peace was restored, and sleep became him. I can never take that back, that smack. I will hate myself forever.

Would I have smacked him and let loose all those other smacks if I had been well? I doubt it. This morning I read a column in the weekend papers where the author was arguing that tough love strategies need to be extended to adults with addictive behaviours that are a plague on society, including internet and sex addicts, workaholics, philanderers, bulimics, and people with depressive disorders who choose to become co-dependent or self-medicate rather than take responsibility for their own condition. She is a columnist, she's paid to have strong opinions. Actually, she was speaking on behalf of the put-upon partners of addicts, and also as someone who has had her own battles with the 'black dog'. What kind of place should tough love have in relationships where someone has depression?

JULY 2005

Dear Susie,

We miss you. Please come home. London does not love you as much as we do.

The whales are swimming past and everyday they flap their tales at us, wondering where you are. Come home.

Love
James, Ulrike, Scarlet and Hunter
xxxxxooooxxxxxxoooxxx

My first 'tough love' act was to ban myself from going to London. I had been to too many conferences and archives and enough was enough. Today I can't even imagine going away for weeks on end as I routinely did then. What on earth was I thinking? Even a night away for work holds no joy now. I must have been sick. Really sick. I apologise. Was it truly my downfall, all this pretending to be a well-honed professional engaged in a flawless recovery from ill-health, or did it honestly keep me sane, or walk me back to sanity? It is too late to know. At the time I didn't feel like I had any alternative but to prove them wrong, my accusers – *I am not a plagiarist look at all I can write you big bad meanies* – but now, today . . . I wish I hadn't missed Hunter's second birthday. I can never have that back.

If I spent as much time on my relationships, friendships and children as I do worrying about staying well, then I would be . . . I know not what. I have an uneasy relationship, based on gross failure, with medication. The most recent attempt at druggery was at least letting me sleep, such a precious commodity. But it was that same group of drugs that had me walking through honey all day, despite dosage modifications. Usually, I don't bother to remember the name of medications. It is an act of wilful neglect. I take drugs to stop me brinking edges through sleeplessness. Otherwise, I hate drugs. I hate them.

Sometimes, however, the best choice for all concerned, the groovy choice, is to shut up and take some. My GP in Melbourne – now my former GP – recently told me to stop moaning about weight gain and concentrate on the higher benefits: keep taking your tablets girl, and you'll get some sleep and be a better mother. I went home and did my own research. It didn't take much to find out that Zyprexa, the drug I'd just been prescribed, had recently been involved in a $690 million lawsuit, settling over 8000 claims filed by people who had presented with diabetes and other diseases that they said were due to their being prescribed the drug. The article said that some doctors have been reluctant to prescribe Zyprexa because they feared they would be sued. The drug company did not expect a second wave of suits, because the label change protects them from people who claim they developed diabetes from taking the drug after 2003. My doctor asked me what I was worried about, the risks were all well documented. I threw the tablets in the bin. I went for a run. I bought of bottle of wine.

Once upon a time, until 1973, homosexuality was listed in the DSM (*Diagnostic Statistical Manual of Mental Disorders*) as a psychiatric condition, pathologised as being in need of treatment. The suggestion was that a disease was a bad thing to have. To be included in the manual, any condition has to be considered both an unlucky thing to have, and possess the potential to be medically treated; these are the criteria for a condition to be a disease. It's not for me to enter into an anti-psychiatry argument. Post-traumatic stress syndrome needed to be included in the DSM, for example, so that the Vietnam vets could be treated on insurance. The history of medicine tells us much about how diseases can be constructed. So what types of mental disorders are natural, and what are constructed? And how well do you think your average GP can buy into that debate?

All classification is a theory-laden exercise. Please don't theorise me out of existence. Or into one I don't endorse, either. Please just wait until psychiatric theory catches up with my lived experience. Just like we have to wait for the metabolic experts to prove clinically what we intuitively know to be true. I will sit here quietly and politely so long as you keep your prescription pads on the desk and away from me. And don't put me on any more crazy registers while you're at it. And, no thanks, a stint in the psych ward does not arouse my curiosities as a writer. Or, I should say, James will stand there being polite, I shall no doubt resort to the odd rant. We've good-copped-bad-copped our way through too many a traffic-jammed Emergency Room not to appreciate the value of that routine. Anyway I will sit here, I promise, feeling as groovy as I can.

LIKE BUTTER IN THE BLACK DOG'S HOUSE

I love that Scottish expression 'like butter in the black dog's house', meaning that something is beyond all recovery. A proverbial saying used to denote what is irrevocably gone, I say it most often to the early-morning-mirror-me, always underslept and often over-graped, looking 10 years older than I did last time I was similarly caught out. I say it to myself because it makes me smile. It makes me remember that I chose the night I lived the night before. I chose the company and the activity and the conversation and even the babies that ship-wrecked any surviving good intentions of an unbroken sleep that remained after my negligent approach to sensible rest had exhausted itself. I chose it over bed and self-help books and, regardless, I chose well if not wisest. I say 'like butter in the black dog's house' because it is nonsensical just like depression and MCADD, which both share a scatological wiring that is beyond my command and sometimes even lucid comprehension. And after I laugh I pretend I want to go for a surf or to yoga or for a run, and after I've thrown the Weetabix around to the right people, I make a choice and I exercise, then I go to work with some smart outfit or other and never without makeup, armed with the lecture and all the marking you did between getting the kids to sleep and sitting down to relax that constituted hour three hundred of the week even though it's only Wednesday, and I pretend I like it. And sometimes I do. Sometimes the goodness of the day sneaks up on me just when I think that surely a bucket of wine with my head in it is much easier than this 'fake fake faking it' stuff.

I believe this about me: if I fall down now I will never get up. So is it better to wear flat heels or have a huge pack of band-aids in your purse? Faking it might be one strategy to get by, but getting your groove back post-diagnosis is a complicated and sometimes never-ending story. What emotional size were you in the first place, when you were well? And is this what one should be aiming for? To re-inhabit old (sometimes haunted) spaces of our former selves? Use what you must. Medication. Clinicians. Family. Friends. To say 'disregard anything or anybody that does not enhance your well-being' is a luxury, and completely disrespectful to the many sufferers of mental illnesses who remain capable enough to play a meaningful role in society, particularly if you have a family to sup-port. Particularly if you know too well the costs of falling down. And this is where expert skills in fakery come into their own. It is not about denial, or self-deception, or idiocy in the face of illness, it is about dignity in measurable grabs. Just because you are having a bad, bad, black dog's butter day, sometimes this does not need to be anybody else's business but your own. Enacting privacy by the concealment of illness through performed wellness is not necessarily the diabolical act of an unwell person, it is sometimes nothing more or less than good manners. And also, perhaps the kindest and most graceful thing you can offer to those around you, who also suffer. The peace that such a decision creates, and the privacy it buys, is often the blessing that I most need on a daily basis. I am not 'over' being ill. The force of life has just moved me beyond it. Is it an imperfection or a line of beauty anyway, illness?

THERE IS MORE THAN ONE KIND OF DARK NIGHT

Sunday. Melbourne University Open Day 2008. We're all there, I forget why. I think the kids love hanging out where daddy works. Soon we'll go to the movies and leave him be, but for now they are running around like typhoons, in university T-shirts way too big for them hooped up with rubber bands, mad little mascots. Ulrike, of course, has much more poise. One of James's students says hi and gives him a copy of a magazine that she picked up for free from the science section – the issue's theme is the brain, and he taught 'Minds and Madness' last semester. The magazine is *Cosmos*. I've never heard of it. It has a very classy short story in it. I promise to read more of the writer's work. Good articles. LSD is making a comeback, apparently, as drug of therapeutic choice. Its use in scientific or medical research is currently prohibited in Australia. Contemporary advocates are arguing that it has unparalleled benefits in the treatment of severe pain, and that its potential to act as an adjunct treatment to psychotherapy should not be ignored. Post-traumatic stress disorders. Substance addiction. Etcetera. Can LSD help us find our sense of self? I thought it was responsible for chasing it away? Who cares! LSD, hooray, old age is starting to look much better. Handling the psyche. Handling experiences. There must be a better balance, somewhere, somehow.

'Mummy do you love butter?'
Scarlet rubs a yellow flower beneath my chin. She believes in magic,
    and omens.
'Yes, you do!'
'What?'
'You have a yellow chin. You like butter.'
'I like you.'
The pollen feels like velvet. Like the soft skin behind her
earlobes.
'I like you too. Can I have a can of coke?'

The children are now hoovering up the free food. More stuff. These scientists are an interesting bunch. National Institute of

Mental Health studies in the US reveal over one year, 5% of 15 000 had experienced hallucinations, like voices talking to them. Only one-third of that group also met the 'crazy criteria' according to psychiatric diagnosis. Boxes, little boxes everywhere. Then there is a graphic article with way too many colour photos of a brain surgery operation. Then an article on the brain and how it transfers memory. This article is so convincing that I start to feel worried that in writing about the past I'm causing a neurological traffic jam: just let them flow unimpeded Susan, you silly woman. Stop being a cattle dog, nipping heels, herding them up for shearing. Because apparently memories aren't stored away in files, they don't have a final resting place, they're very dynamic. According to this expert. The dumping of information can overwrite existing memories on the cortex. This sounds dangerous. I decide to stop writing my book. I thought the life of the brain was too mysterious for science, I thought it belonged to philosophy. I need to read more. I get it wrong, all the time.

The semester is writing its Dear John letter to all of our sleep-less nights, rendering such devotion and anxiety as what it is – old rock, now pebbled, just a part of the long, wet river. All that is left is a temptingly combustible pile of marking, and some apologies to make to I've forgotten whom. And about what? Surely my negli-gence as mother and daughter and friend. It's just a job, and a not very well paid one, which makes the double time that we all put into this game some kind of nonsense. I forget the time. Nervous exhaustion has left me powerless, and locks me to my ergonomic chair as though I am naked, strapped in, awaiting an examination for I know not what.

I pick a whole pile of correspondence and other papers, my 'LIST D priority', up off the floor and throw it in the bin. Not even across the room in the recycling bin, it has to be this one, this clos-est one, damp and messy with forgotten tofu pies and coffee and apple cores and tissues. So that I might not be tempted to retrieve the work, to answer letters, to finish poems so bad they deserve dumping, not the resuscitation that would have blued them further. I turn, instead, to a file that does matter. Priority A. From my desk drawer I take out the photos, and I breathe in the pictures of the babies – big, yoga breaths full of them – one day I will suffocate them with my deep sucking need.

Inside the red folder, crayoned with 'special considerations', is an outstanding claim for just that: special consideration. It is not unusual to have students with mental health problems. Or unusual for them to have spells where they're unable to work, documented by their doctors, requesting consideration that they hand in work late, later, and that understanding be exercised. It is – what is it? – paperwork. But of course this is a big fat lie. Each case that comes across my desk is me. It is a me that tripped harder, or fell softer, or has more hands to hold, or less veins left to mine. It is a me that I wished I had been, one that life took pause from, and spelled, whilst young. Here I am heading for menopause and coming out about a mental health problem that frankly I don't know why more people didn't notice. Or say something about. Am I the only woman in my family to have been to this place? Women's business it may be, but the way I've lived my life, it seems to be nobody's business but mine to deal with, that's how lonely it has felt. I could howl 'unloved', but what a wolf cry that would be, as I know I have been. Loved.

In my forties, that's all, but that's more than old enough to sit around on the beach or in an English garden in the almost summer rain and talk of old age and care and how we shall live those last years of our life. My ex-husband talks of buying property in Italy with friends, pooling life savings, hiring a full-time nurse. Other friends rabbit on about reinventing the nuclear family, neglecting to note they have spent their whole life so far avoiding said family – disregarding, disrespecting, dodging alimony payments for – but suddenly this notion, this wish for family grows into a recognisable logic as the heart starts its biggest hurting. Others buy into retirement villas that can accommodate their grand piano. Lots more just sit around drinking too much, petrified, jabbing in comments about 'what superannuation?', and 'clever you with your equity wealth'. And me?

I wish this. My children to be free, and strong enough to say no to all the things that have yessed me sick all my life. To feel once again the love that circulated in my life before depression brought me down. To be able to write, forever, and to have Friday/Freitag as my favourite metaphor for life. That the day, this one day at least, is 'free'. And if I must be without the wet hammer kisses of children and their unbidden love as they grow and go, and the conversation and touch of him, my husband, if we don't make it, then I want to grow old with people that I don't have to apologise to all the time for being weird, or worry myself raw around sensible, happy people who jerk at my strange utterances and brittle ambitions, all devoted to the vanity of the galaxy within, which one day, thankfully, will simply ember out. And I ask for no special consideration, and will not. Except this: the wish that we could all take better pause to ponder the postmodernity of madness, its cause and effect, without forever calculating the cost.

I like the stillness of good health, its calm breeze. Here I am. Me with my cyclothymic moods and an invisible black dog in the boot of the car. If I had to write a list of things that define me most, 'tired' would be at the top. Nothing unique about that. I'm not sure where 'writer' would appear. 'Mother' is the page this entire list would be written on, and turn the page over; there I am again, 'wife, beloved'. A question that a lot of people might wonder about is, does 'mentally ill' make this list, does it rank? Or, if they were really worried, does 'suicidal' write itself an invitation? With someone like me, whom medical practitioners classify as having 'a significant background history', how revealing can a 'cyclothymic personality style' really be? In terms of self-revelation, it has meant an enormous amount to me, particularly in making sense of what has been. It has also helped me locate a belief that the future may be different than I had imagined. Care. It is about care, and its context. Just because I may not describe any suicidal ideation, or reveal any evidence of psychosis (though, I ask you, where is truth if not in poetry?), this secret may be better explained in terms of resolve rather than honesty.

My only message then, is that I was best understood when my writing was (finally, properly) read, and when the right fisherman caught the narrative of what had really happened. And reading is a complicated act. I speak whole worlds of lies for an overcrowded universe of reasons. My GP finally had access to what was really going on after it was all over, when he read the collection of poems. It wasn't too late for me. But it often is for a lot of people. Having babies is meant to be one of the happiest things in life. How I wish I could have my time again, to feed them and love them free from despair.

We all of us live our lives with less aplomb than we'd like. Who sells us these lies of perfection that riptide us away into Prozac Nations anyway? It doesn't need to be like that, chasing perfect. It just needs to be better. All that breathing practise in antenatal classes was a waste of time. I needed my oxygen most when it was all over. Now I can breathe again. And most of all I like to breathe deeply of the top of my babies' heads. I like to hold them in my arms whenever they let me, and breathe them in. Because for oh so long I never did. And I drop them at school and nursery, and I drive to the university, and I sit in my office before class and I write to them. To still my heart.

'The Scarlet series of true belief'

The stress underwent its adrenalin transformation
when her lip suddenly curled as I offered my breast,
panic became me, and although we were two blocks
away, in A&E, within 10 minutes, her coma lasted
a thousand times longer than that, it had its own
smoke and smell and they linger still in my blood.

Jumpoline.
Footyball.
Eleventeen.
Baby Anabelle
did a smell

I've seen I've seen I've seen
her live and grow, post diagnosis,
but she remains forever grey in the
retina between me and reality. I pray,
and take too many photos, in case
the smoke finds a way to escape.
Please, draw me a person.

And then I put my poems away. I have no photos on my desk any more. Only pens. I don't want strangers, students, seeing them, my children. And yet here I am, telling you everything.

Last week 'Daddy' came home from five weeks away in London town. He's writing a good book, he had to go away, but seeing his girls, and his Mum and Dad and brother and *god what do we leave behind?* was the better blessing. Here, home in Australia, he had missed a 5th birthday party and a ride in a seaplane and the school holidays and moving into our new home and a visit from Germany from Matthias, and all the tears and love in between. But, gloriously, James got back just in time for the opening of *The Dark Knight*, the latest Batman movie that despite its adult rating I had promised to take Hunter to as a belated birthday treat. He extracted this promise from me when he was still four. Outside Melbourne University kindergarten is a huge advertising billboard, and it won that argument. So off we went. The IMAX theatre at the Melbourne Museum was then the world's largest screen. I know this to be true – the information is ensconced permanently on a marbled floor. There seemed to be plenty of other people there in that sold-out session on a rainy winter Sunday, ignoring censorship advice, but most of the little kids had left crying, with annoyed parents, fairly early on. I think this is maybe because that big screen really does make you feel 'dizzy sick'. We stayed. It was fabulous, I spent the whole time watching the kids watching Batman. Afterwards, Hunter's 5-year-old criticism declared that the movie is really all about the Joker, and that he's not really dead, and that Batman will have to fight him again. One day real soon. Scarlet thinks it is a love story and will not believe that Batman's true love Rachel was blown up. She too will rise again, Scarlet insisted, probably in a wedding dress. She's six. She likes on-screen kissing. My students, if they did indeed have one, wouldn't offer an opinion in today's class. They were mostly still all upset about Heath. Me, I thought it was all about chaos theory. I don't know what James thought; he was jetlagged and had a nap. Ulrike was away up north, surfing in Lennox Head, her Papa over from Germany and duly impressed. School seems irrelevant temporarily. She's still 10. She went to see the new Abba movie instead. Harm in all its harmless cinematic glory. Thank god for goodness. We, all of us, have seen the insides of too many hospitals, with their shiny chaos and black magic. Maybe that's why Scarlet and Hunter were unfazed by the goodie-turned-baddie missing half a face. They've seen it all before.

WHAT ARE YOU LIKE?

If you have ever had a mental health 'difficulty', then sometimes your most legitimate longing is for that time in your life to be forgotten. Unremembered. Vanished. Vamoosed. Disappeared. But, you can never be unmarked. Can you? Isn't an erased tattoo nothing more than a double scarring? Two traumatic events, marking and unmarking. If I had a wish to spend, would I really wish this dark time of my life away?

Babar the King is a bedtime reading favourite of Hunter's. Babar builds his perfect colonial society in a found paradise, and one and all in the kingdom are living faithful, true, and happy lives, which they celebrate one day with a glorious carnival. On this same day, the beloved old lady of the kingdom is bitten by a snake, and fire wreaks havoc in his adviser's house. Thus, two of Babar's most cherished friends are hospitalised, their lives in the balance.

That night, for the first time ever, the King is visited by the figure of Misfortune. Misfortune is, of course, as ever, in the guise of a hideous old woman. 'Shoo, shoo', Babar says to his dreams. But, no. Misfortune has brought her friends along. Despair. Cowardice. Indolence. Ignorance. Laziness. Fear. All of them meteoring their way across the dark universe to invade Babar's perfect world. But hark! His nightmare turns to dream, heralded by a visitation of angels; well, white elephants with wings to be precise. Misfortune is chased away from the kingdom by Happiness, and good angel-elephant allies: Goodness, Hope, Health, Intelligence, Joy, Learning, Patience, Work, Perseverance, and Courage. Not forgetting, of course, Love. Our favourite is Courage, for she carries a giant sword in her trunk. Back in the real world, Babar's friends recover. The wicked snake and the demon fire achieve no triumph. Babar and all subjects, from that day on, lived in peace and happiness. Because they never lost heart, you see. Their collective will was the hero of their story.

Literary criticism, or drawing strength and wisdom from story, has always worked for me when I've felt down. Text, and its secret, storied heart, has comforted so many, so often through time. Solace in the words of the Bible, and so on. But, like Hunter, I am never completely sold on 'salvation', on elephants flying through the air dressed like choir children, particularly when the baddies seem to have the better costumes, with a touch of 'pirate hip' about them. The power of narrative to save or heal can be a dubious claim, with that mass-manufactured feel of the greeting card industry about it. I do believe in the therapeutic potential of writing, and reading, but when you're truly 'down', sometimes I think there is nothing for it but to just be down, and not to insist on the angel of Words, or any angel, to fly you away from all harm. Perhaps I say this purely from my own experiential viewpoint, which was one of muteness, of being unable to read or write when I was most ill. Who is to say, though, that this retreat from 'intelligence', if you like, was not a necessary part of recovery? Perhaps also, it is because my favourite part of the Babar book is when all the little elephants sing the 'Song of the elephants', as a surprise. The words are all nonsense. There is a note, explaining: the song is an old song, the song of the mammoths, in fact, and not a living soul knows what the words mean.

Words and writing may help you stay healthy, and do indeed keep me from falling into harm's way again, but two things, for what they're worth: it was my children's songs that sang me back to life, their songs with all their secret, mammoth magic. And, even if that wish ever did come my way, I would never ask to be thus unmarked, to have never heard their song.

CAUTIONARY TALES

Peter Porter's beautiful and cautionary poem 'Old friends' worries about the virtues of writers writing, for example, 'spacious memoir[s]', despite their elegance. 'Is it right that we spike our life like this?' he asks. While Peter himself made his own decisions about this, famously returning an advance to his publisher for a promised autobiography, it is a different thing, a different animal, poetry. Poetry is the kingdom wherein permission is best granted for writers to be 'caught by their trade', as he put it, and reveal all. I couldn't agree more. When I have been most worried about revealing myself, and in so doing causing harm to others, by betraying them with my memories, my stories, my 'talk' about them, I have to surrender, caught. For there is no more weaponry in this little book than in any of my published poems. So all my 'sorries' began a long time ago. Or should have. It is the business of poetry to scream. But here, in the confessional genre of memoir, I find the hush of writing far more painful. No matter how 'awful' the stuff of my poetry from this period may be, no matter how autobiographical its impulse, it is fiction.

And this, dear reader, is a true tale. Told by a woman who cried the flood of Noah when her baby died in the second trimester, lost forever to the incinerator of University College London Hospital, choking Bloomsbury with my ashen grief, strangling my marriage. It is the true tale of that same woman, who, baby after baby, was stolen away from happiness, molecule by honeyed molecule, until I turned myself inside out, hunting all through London Town for Wendy Darling to stitch my shadow back, so that I might fly home to Neverland. Full of all the lost children. Mine. My lost babies, who 'had to walk side by little step with me through the docks / and dikes of suicide alley . . .' – this was their infant journey.

When I am so old that I make my children cry because I can no longer recall them when they come to visit me, I would very much like them to know that I had lived a life that warranted a poem, or a song, or two. And, despite the costs, that it was worth it. For me. In case they're wondering, while they're busy paying for all my excessive geriatric medical care because I used to eat magic mushroom sandwiches with honey in high school and therein lies the tragedy. But really, most of all, my legitimate longing is that they know this: that when Misfortune visited me, and took me away, and broke me down, she never touched that part of me that knew their love. No matter what mad songs or otherwise I sang, or may sing. As Peter Porter says in that same poem, 'We're packed too tight/to trust ourselves in this existence'. Amen. But – there is something in writing about the past, about lived life, beyond poetry, that I do trust. Maybe it is the historian in me, with my unfashionable desire for the *wie es eigentlich gewesen* school of history, to know everything *as it actually was*, that quest for steadfast, trustworthy revelation.

Impossible: I was there, but I was not. Despite the perils of writing a memoir, there are worse kinds of suicide than that of unseemly revelation. Reading memoirs has left me with more discriminating appetites, hopefully trustworthy ones, and a yearning to say something more testimonial about existence and our crushed abilities to know ourselves. So. That's enough on longing. I write this for my children, this memoir, this shadow narrative of those poems, and offer it in all its tight packaging. It is a story to sardine my way out of trouble, whilst singing a song of love to those whose siren kept me alive.

And in this narrative, there we all are.